Transform

Books by Lori Ann King

Come Back Strong
Balanced Wellness After Surgical Menopause

Wheels to Wellbeing
A Practical Self-Care Guide to Living a More Balanced Life

Courses by Lori Ann King

Balanced Wellness During Menopause

Books By Jim and Lori Ann King

Raging Love
An Athlete's Journey to Self-Validation and Purpose (2022)

Transform

**BUILDING THE MINDSET TO CHANGE
YOUR BODY AND YOUR LIFE**

Lori Ann King

Gunnison Press
LAS CRUCES, NM

Lori Ann King/Gunnison Press
Email: info@loriannking.com
Website: www.LoriAnnKing.com

Book Layout ©2018 BookDesignTemplates.com
Copy editing by FirstEditing.com
Cover design by Gus Yoo
Cover Photo by Brandon Tigrett

Ordering Information: Quantity sales. Special discounts are available on quantity purchases by corporations, associations, libraries, and others. For details, contact bulkorders@loriannking.com.

Library of Congress Control Number 9780999542347

Transform/ Lori Ann King. —1st ed.

ISBN 978-0-9995423-4-7

For Jim, who told me I could change anything about myself except the length of my bones.

Contents

Acknowledgments

I acknowledge with love, gratitude, and kindness:

Jim. I first trusted you with my outsides, as you helped build proportion into my physique. You later trusted me with your insides when nutrition and weight loss became a matter of life and death.

To the finalists who came before me, thank you for paving the way.

For the finalists who came after me and future finalists, keep sharing your truth. Someone needs to hear your story.

For my finalists, you pick me up when I'm feeling down, you celebrate every victory with me, and you continue to inspire me with your passion, grace, and unconditional love.

For the sixteen-week transformation challenge, thank you for the accountability, support, cash, coupons, swag, and Costa Rica. Pura Vida.

I thank my editor, Michael at First Editing.

To Gus Yoo, thank you for another beautiful cover design.

Introduction

"PLEASE WELCOME TO THE stage, Lori King!"

The music thundered and the crowd roared as I took my place amongst fourteen other finalists from a sixteen-week transformation challenge. We all cheered and high-fived, many of us with tears in our eyes, mostly from joy, but also from the sheer overwhelm of the crowd, as well as the memories of how hard we had worked to get there.

It had been a month since we had each received the phone call that would forever change our lives. Since then, there had been Zoom calls and Marco Polos where we all quickly got to know each other. In the days prior to being on stage, there were dinners and photoshoots once we had all gathered in Phoenix, Arizona at a New Year's Kick-Off event. We knew each other's stories, family members, and dreams. The challenge brought us together. Many of us—the girls especially—would stay together, communicating daily or at least weekly on Marco Polo, forever bonded as friends and "chosen" members of our family and tribe.

It had been a long journey for each of us. I was the "veteran" of the group, having participated in thirteen previous sixteen-week challenges.

After my first challenge in 2014, I was selected as an honorable mention. Shortly after this victory my husband, Jim, joined me. At the completion of every challenge, we enrolled again, each time waiting and hoping for a phone call saying we were selected as a finalist. Month after month, year after year, the call didn't come.

Until one summer day in July of 2017: Jim got the call. After seven completed challenges he was selected as a finalist. On the stage, in front of thousands of people, he was chosen as that year's runner-up, winning $10,000 and redefining what age 65 is supposed to look like in terms of health and fitness.

It was another two years before I got the phone call, making us one of three United States couples to both become finalists. It was worth the wait.

At the time of this writing, combined we have completed over 40 sixteen-week challenges. We have more than twenty-four years of experience combined in transforming our bodies and our minds. Add in Jim's powerlifting career and years as a personal trainer and it's more like 50 years. We have over 100 years of experience combined as athletes.

We are writers, authors, and bloggers. Jim is a national champion in powerlifting and I am an Amazon best-selling author. We've had success as road cyclists and bodybuilders, in business, and in love.

But success is never constant nor is it a straight line. There are peaks and valleys, highs and lows, and health and wellness ebb and flow with the seasons of our lives.

I've survived abuse, divorce, a five-plus-year battle with chronic idiopathic hives, and surgical menopause. I've been told I was too skinny and felt I could not change my body's genetic predispositions, until Jim told me I could change anything except the length of my bones. Talk about empowering.

Jim has survived physical limitations, abuse, bullying, racial prejudice, oppression, divorce, disappointments, a 95% blockage in the "widowmaker" artery of his heart, surgery in both knees and one of his shoulders, two foot surgeries, and prostate cancer and surgery to remove his prostate.

We struggled through the Covid-19 Pandemic, experiencing loneliness, the loss of two income streams, and a 2,300+ mile move across the country, all while dealing with a cancer diagnosis and treatment plan amidst a season of self-isolation.

There are times we don't feel worthy and times when we seek comfort in food. Time and time again it is our mindset that gets us out of a funk, propels us forward, and allows us to live life more abundantly.

As we've studied and lived a life focused on health and wellbeing, we've discovered that wellness is a three-sided structure that involves exercise, nutrition, and mindset. This book is not about the specific diet or exercise that you should follow to reach success. I won't teach you how to count macros or give you specific workouts. Your success in health and wellness and your compliance with exercise and nutrition depends on your mental strength and resilience, and that is what this book is about.

I am writing to dispel the myths or lies that you tell yourself as to why you can't have success: you're too old, you're too young, you're divorced, you've been abused, you're menopausal, you're too skinny, you're overweight, you have a disease or illness, or simply, you don't feel worthy. I've been there. I've dealt with these lies in my own life and if I can overcome them, so can you.

My goal is to empower you to become the healthiest, happiest, most successful version of yourself that you can—whatever that means to you. As part of my mission to inspire you to live life more abundantly, I'm sharing the top tips, rules, and mindsets that I've embraced on my journey to success. It's MY turn to pay it forward and it's YOUR turn to create your own success story as well as your own happiness.

Understanding Wellness

Wellness can be defined as the quality or state of being healthy in body and mind, especially as the result of deliberate effort. In its basic form, think of wellness as a triangle comprised of three key components: exercise, nutrition, and mental strength. The physical component of wellness is often the easiest to measure, but it's not the only component to a healthy life.

As a wellness consultant married to a personal trainer and sports nutritionist, I have found that exercise and nutrition are fairly easy to implement. Exercise is added to a person's schedule to include cardiovascular, strength training, and flexibility. If you are not already active, I put on my detective cap and find out if there was anything in your childhood that you loved to do, such as ride a bike or play volleyball. Next, I explore ways to bring that activity and passion back into your life.

For nutrition, Jim and I partner with an extraordinary health and wellness company that provides nutritional systems that work to fuel the body for athletics, weight loss, graceful aging, performance, energy, and an overall healthy lifestyle. We show people how to turn their everyday healthy food money into an income-producing asset. We offer nutrition backed by cutting-edge science, guided by a scientific advisory board with third-party clinical studies. Our products are soy-free and gluten-free, with dairy-free options. Whether you follow a keto, paleo, 40 / 30 / 30, plant-based, Mediterranean, or alien lifestyle, our products and systems can fit into your diet and make living a healthy lifestyle simpler and more manageable.

The caveat for both exercise and nutrition is compliance. And that's where the tricky part comes in. Your greatest success can be determined by whether or not you survive many crappy days, where you move away from your goals while being diligent with the good days that move you toward your goals. Your success in health and wellness boils down to that third piece of the triangle: your mental strength. And your mental strength determines whether you will be compliant with exercise and nutrition.

So, why is wellness so hard to achieve?

The truth is, many people are not willing to do the second part of wellness: the deliberate effort, specifically in regard to mental strength. They are not willing to make wellness a top priority or are not ready to change.

Our mind is just like our muscles: when we focus on building muscles and training them with daily consistent action, they grow. If we stop training, they atrophy. When it comes to our mental state, what we think about, we get more of. It's like when you are thinking about buying a Jeep, and suddenly every other car you see on the road is a Jeep. Or if you or someone you love is pregnant, and you start seeing pregnant women everywhere you go. This is the power of your mind and its ability to focus.

In the case of weight loss for a healthy lifestyle, something as simple as saying "I want to lose weight" or "I don't want to be overweight" can have devastating consequences. Your subconscious hears "wanting, losing, and overweight" and gives you more of that. This not only leaves you always wanting but in the rare case where you do lose weight, you gain it back because it is ingrained in your subconscious that "what is lost wants to be found."

A better statement is "I release weight with ease." Now your subconscious focuses on releasing and ease. Focus your thoughts on what you want (health, leanness, strength), not on what you don't want (losing or being overweight or underweight).

Data vs Emotion

While speaking to a friend who was on a quest to release twenty pounds, I asked about her workouts. There was a pause, and I could almost hear the self-loathing in her sigh and the feeling of somehow being "less than" because she wasn't working out as much as she'd like to, or "should" be according to her own or someone else's standard.

To me, my question—and the answer—was just data; data that I needed to coach and advise her on nutrition.

To her, there was an emotion tied to it. But emotion is better utilized when attached to something positive and goal-oriented, as opposed to failure or something negative. Diet, nutrition, fitness, exercise, and resolutions are all buzzwords in the health and wellness industry. What I have found is that words like diet and resolutions leave us feeling "less than." Like we haven't reached success yet. That we are somehow not enough or not worthy of health and success.

What if we were to take the emotion out of it? What if we were to look at things like scale weight, body measurements, and before photos simply as data; as information we track?

So often, when Jim and I coach people toward a healthier lifestyle, we encounter resistance over this tracking process that includes scale weight, body measurements, and before and after photos. To us, it's just data that we use to adjust and tweak to get you your best results.

We don't look at you with judgment. We look at you as human beings on a path, a journey—just like we are—toward being your healthiest, best self. Toward building more consistency into your healthy lifestyle. You are worthy. You are good enough. You deserve to look and feel your best.

Regardless of the size, shape, or condition of your body, it is a temple. Stop beating it up. Stop beating yourself up.

- When you love yourself and your body, you will no longer talk about going on a diet. You'll talk about living a healthy lifestyle. The reason so many diets fail is the mindset going into it. If you plan on a diet or a quick fix where you will eat a healthy diet and exercise for 30 days, and then go back to your current eating plan or lifestyle, then you are setting yourself up to fail. Healthy living is a process and a journey of daily consistent action that you can maintain.

- When you love yourself and your body, you'll look at the scale weight as data and a numerical reflection of your relationship with gravity. This data provides feedback as to whether or not you are on the right path, or if you require an adjustment. It is a number that reflects information from the prior day or days.

- When you love yourself and your body, you'll look at food as fuel. You'll eat foods with optimum nutrients that will help you live life to the fullest.

If, however, you beat yourself up and don't show yourself self-love, then you'll experience guilt and shame, and ultimately you'll find it easier to abuse and sabotage yourself, your body, and your health and wellness goals.

Think for a minute. When you beat yourself up or feel sorry for yourself, isn't it easier to grab a box of cookies, a bag of potato chips, or a bottle of wine, put on your PJs and curl up in front of the television?

A healthy mindset learns to transform emotions from something associated with failure to something associated with achieving steps toward your goals. Set a fixed non-food reward for success and celebrate the small victories. Show yourself self-love for your achievements.

When you love yourself, you give yourself the nutrients and exercise your body requires as fuel, to energize you through life as an athlete, wife, husband, mom, dad, partner, caretaker, employee, boss, leader, and contributor. When you love yourself, you put self-love in action toward a healthy lifestyle.

Love Your Body and Want to Change It

There are a multitude of reasons for why you might want to change your body. And those reasons may change and evolve over time.

In my thirties, I dreamed of having a healthy digestive system, better focus, balanced hormones, and a lean physique. I upgraded my nutrition and lost 21 pounds, 27 inches, and 9% body fat. I felt Ah-Ma-Zing.

Satisfied with my results, I set a new goal. I dreamed of being a beast on my bike. With my new power-to-weight ratio, enhanced nutrition, and a lot of conditioning, within two years I posted the second fastest speed by a woman on the five-mile Bear Mountain Climb in New York's Hudson Valley.

I still wasn't finished. I set my sights on building a strong, muscular body with a killer set of abs. I optimized my nutrition still further, increased my calories to 2,600 per day, and moved my focus from training on my bike to lifting weights in the gym. The following year, I received an honorable mention in a sixteen-week transformation challenge. I set my sights on my next goal: to become a finalist in that same contest.

But an unexpected surgery plunged me into full-blown surgically induced menopause. It stole much of my progress away. My doctors told me that gaining weight was to be expected. It was part of aging. Suddenly, my goal became about reclaiming my body and my vitality.

With a community of support and world-class nutrition, I once again achieved my goal. I became healthier, more confident, and more balanced than I had ever been. To this day I feel vibrant, energized, and alive as I live my life more abundantly in my body, mind, and life. It took a little longer than expected, but I eventually achieved my next goal of becoming a finalist.

Jim's goals changed over time as well. At 40 he became a powerlifting national champion. But after achieving this elite status, he didn't have a plan in place for "What's next?" He stopped lifting but continued to eat as if he was training, which caused the weight to pile on.

By the time he reached 50 years old, he felt "old, overweight, and less than." Then, his own personal health scare, combined with his poor family medical history, had his doctors telling him that he needed to change his lifestyle and his diet, and improve his overall health.

Jim used that health scare to fuel his desire for change. He lost 40 pounds and 10 inches off his waist, and at 65 years old, he became an ambassador for healthy aging. Now approaching 70, he has survived a cardiovascular scare and prostate cancer. He continues to sever the link between age and value. He is not measured by a calendar, the number of rotations around the sun, or a number associated with some paradigm of a progressive state of decline. Today, Jim measures his worth by how he feels, his energy level, and his success in reaching his goals and sustaining athletic accomplishments. (You can read more of his story in our book, *Raging Love: An Athlete's Journey to Self-Validation and Purpose* (2022).)

Jim and I are far from perfect. We are human. There are times when we are more fit and times when we are less fit. There are times we eat poorly and times we follow a healthy diet consistently. I have been 20 pounds overweight and frustrated with how my clothes fit. Jim has been 40 pounds overweight with concerns over his morbidity and quality of his life. There are times we work hard to look and feel our best, and there are times we slack off on our efforts, and we often look and feel the results of that.

But just to be clear, there is one thing that remains consistent in our life: whatever state we are in physically, most of the time we love ourselves for who we are. In those times we may become disappointed in ourselves, we strive even harder to practice self-love while focusing on building a strong mindset, knowing we have the power to change what we don't like.

Our lives are constantly under construction; there is always something to improve. We strive to improve and change because we love ourselves, knowing that we can love our bodies and want to change them.

Sticks and Stones

As a child Jim grew up being told over and over again, "sticks and stones can break my bones, but words can never hurt me."

He grew up as a very short "nerd," who moved every three years to a new school system due to his father's military career. This did not get him the attention he craved as a young child. All the other kids his age were bigger and faster. He was the shortest person in every grade until ninth grade, when he was finally taller than one girl in his class. he was bullied. He got called weak; a faggot; a nigger.

But, no worries. He was one of the smartest kids, adored by his teachers, and after all, "sticks and stones can break my bones, but words can never hurt me."

In tenth grade, he shot up six inches and bloomed into a 98-pound young man. At 5'6", he entered the arena of high school wrestling where he thrived. He was popular. He was friends with fellow varsity teammates. He achieved athletic excellence. And to top it off, he had a really cool girlfriend. Suddenly, nobody was calling him names.

But in eleventh grade, Jim's father returned from Vietnam with Post Traumatic Stress Disorder (PTSD). He had been physically hard on Jim his entire life. Now, he was beating Jim. He gave him quite a large dosage of "sticks and stones."

The funny thing is, Jim doesn't remember the pain of the beatings. But he remembers the feeling of every word that his father said. His harsh words implanted a blueprint in Jim's subconscious that caused him to struggle for over 20 years. In his forties, with the help of four years of therapy, he finally dealt with freeing himself of this pain through a few simple laws.

Law of forgiveness: Jim chose to forgive his father so that there were no feelings of anger or resentment interfering with his happiness or ability to love and serve others.

Law of substitution: Instead of focusing on toxic memories and feelings of unworthiness, Jim focused on life goals. This led him to win a national championship in powerlifting, setting a national record in the deadlift in the process.

Law of practice: For over five years he worked out five times a week, without missing a single training session, with two different world champions and a USA national championship team.

Law of dual thought: Regardless of how much pain he endured, Jim told himself that life was great. His pain was simply a strong indicator that he was changing and morphing into the person he was required to be to be the best in the world.

Law of growth: For 13 years Jim was either at the gym lifting or thinking about the next time he would be at the gym lifting. It led him to strive and work to improve and succeed in all aspects of life, as it was important to feel great in order to be great.

Law of relaxation: Recovery in athletics is all about the ability to relax your mind so that your body follows. What you do to recover from work efforts is just as important as what you do during work efforts, and this allows you to put everything into the next efforts 100%.

The truth is, words are important, for they shape your thoughts, mold your beliefs, and influence your actions, which determine your results. Only you can choose what you desire to believe, what you let influence your feelings, what you dwell on, what you act on, and what you determine your pathway to your future to be.

Sticks and stones can break your bones and words can shape the future you. Choose wisely what you desire to believe, grasp onto, and internalize. And be careful what you say to yourself.

Hiding, Hurting, and Healing Through Transformation

Weight loss and body changes are more than just a physical experience. Transformations run so much deeper, to the emotional, psychological, and spiritual. As you lose weight, layers upon layers of hiding come off. It's a physical process. But it's also emotional.

Statistics say that one out of five people has been abused. I dare say it's higher. Many years ago, I was in a car headed toward New York City with three of my girlfriends. All of us were around age 40. Jessica had recently discovered or remembered abuse from her past. Maria chimed in with compassion, having had her own post-abuse fallout. Jade looked at me and said, "Well, Lori. Are you going to make it four for four?"

Every single one of us had been abused.

Maybe that's not exactly true for you. But it's more than likely that you've been hurt at some point in your life by your mother, father, sister, brother, cousin, aunt, teacher, friend, lover, co-worker, or pastor. Somewhere along the line, we've all been hurt.

And what do humans do when they hurt?

They hide.

You hide in your body, your clothes, your love, your relationships, your church, and your job. You stop making eye contact. Your smile fades. Your eyes lose their sparkle.

You hide behind a computer. You cover up your light. You play small. You stop dreaming. You forget your purpose. You become lukewarm, without passion.

When you hide, you feel shame. You gain weight because maybe somehow you'll be safer there. People won't be attracted to you or abuse you. People won't hurt you

If you've been hurt, if you are hiding, I'm asking you to come out and play. To shine your light. To stop playing small. To live your best life in your best body.

When I transformed my body, when I released the weight, I was also able to shed some baggage and some past hurts. There will be more work to do, however, changing the physical can become a catalyst and if you let it, it can become the match that sets the flames of fire and passion that is your life aglow. And you will see shifts in relationships, confidence, career, finances, and more. If you let it. But you have to do the work.

YOUR TURN

What myths or lies have you believed as to why you can't achieve success?

_____

_____

To successfully transform your body and /or change your life, your wellness goal must be extremely important and a top priority. How important is it to you that you accomplish your goals?

_____

Are you willing to change your beliefs about why you have not been successful?   YES / NO

Are you willing to give up your excuses and work toward becoming the healthiest, happiest, most successful version of yourself that you can be?
                                                                            YES / NO

What do you love about your body?

_____

_____

What would you like to change or improve about your body?

CHAPTER 1

_____

_____

What and Why

MY INITIAL GOAL WHEN I joined the sixteen-week transformation challenge was to win. I wanted the $25k prize for winning as well as the title. In our book, *Raging Love: An Athlete's Journey to Self-Validation and Purpose* (2022), Jim wrote about my need to win:

> *When Lori first started cycling, I introduced her to some elite athletes to guide and nurture her. Shauna was competing in the duathlon at a national and world-class level. Laura was enjoying huge success as a nationally ranked Ironman Triathlete. These women were competing at their highest potential and had already achieved greatness. In addition, I was a national champion in powerlifting. I could see Lori wanted something of her own. She had the drive and determination of a pit bull.*
> *In her forties by now, many would say she had missed her prime for achieving success in sports, especially as a beginner cyclist. But we both knew she just had to find her niche.*

As a runner for over twenty years, I always felt I was putting forth a half-assed effort. I ran more or less to stay in shape and maintain my weight as well as for the social aspect of chatting with friends. I ran and raced everything from a two-mile Shamrock run that ended with green bagels and beer, to a half and full-length marathon (13.1 and 26.2 miles respectively). I achieved moderate success, running a sub-four-hour marathon.

When I switched to the bike, I felt like I could fly. I played around with racing, but knew that rising up through the bike categories to pro would require years of dedication and traveling every weekend to race. It would be my sole focus for years. I wasn't sure I had that long-term dedication.

And if I'm honest with myself, I had a fear of racing at high speed in close quarters with other cyclists.

In the gym, I felt strong. With the sixteen-week transformation challenge, beneath my goal of winning and earning a title, there was the desire for my outsides to match my insides. Since the challenge was only sixteen weeks, I knew I could set a short-term goal, get in shape, and look as strong as I felt. Maybe I could even earn the title of finalist and a little prize money.

By the time I reached my thirteenth challenge, my goals had changed. It was no longer about being a certain size or weight or being in top physical condition. Having overcome a major setback of illness (endometriosis), surgery, and the surgical menopause that came after, I wanted to prove to myself that I could come back strong as a post-menopausal woman. I wanted to inspire others in the process, letting the world know that success is never a straight line. It's always a journey that is filled with peaks and valleys. And that anyone, regardless of their age, medical history, or other trials, can turn their setbacks, challenges, and obstacles into comebacks, victories, and lessons learned.

Define Your Goal

Healthy can mean different things to different people. It's important to know what healthy means to you personally. And keep in mind that wellness can mean different things during different seasons of your life. At one time, it may mean being able to perform or compete athletically. Another season may be about achieving a healthy weight. And still, another could be having the energy to keep up with your kids or grandkids.

Define what healthy means to you. Not what other people, magazines or society says is healthy. What do you want as part of a healthy lifestyle? Here are a few ideas:

- Weight loss or gain (yes, some people struggle to put on or maintain a healthy weight)
- Strength
- Flexibility
- Good quality sleep
- Increased energy
- Better digestion
- Improved performance as an athlete, musician, writer, or in life in general
- Rewarding relationships—with God, yourself, your partner, friends, family
- Financial fitness
- Multiple streams of income

- Building a passive stream of income
- Mental focus and clarity
- Emotional stability
- Graceful aging
- Setting a new personal record (PR) in your sport

As you explore what healthy means to you, be sure to:

- **Write It Down.**
  Whatever healthy means to you, be sure to write down your own personal definition. Include your health goals and dreams. Put it in an area that you will see it every day, such as on the refrigerator, the bathroom mirror, or near your calendar.
- **Be Specific.**
  Make sure not only that you set goals, but that you set *clear* and *specific* goals. This will keep you on track and give you a standard to know when you achieve them. For example, "I will eat a healthy breakfast meal replacement shake every day" vs "I will begin to eat healthier" or "I will move my body for twenty minutes five times this week" vs "I will get to the gym more."
- **Give Yourself a Deadline.**
  Without a deadline, it's easy to procrastinate or get stuck in the "someday" circle where you start to feel you are on a never-ending hamster wheel. Make sure it's realistic. If you have gained twenty pounds since your last physical, don't expect to release it all the first month.
- **Start with the End in Mind.**
  With every sixteen-week challenge, I mark the end date on my calendar. Then, I work backward, labeling each week with the number of weeks I have left. If my goal is to release 16 pounds, then my weekly goal is one pound per week. One pound per week sounds much more manageable than 16 pounds.
- **Start Now.**
  You don't have to have one last binge or eat all of your favorite foods over the next few days. You don't have to wait for Monday, or the first of the month, or until you feel like it. You can choose to simply start today. Start now.
- **Assess and Pivot.**
  Wherever you are at the time of your deadline, make sure to evaluate and assess how well you did at accomplishing your original, specific goal by your deadline. Did you reach your goal in the time frame you said you would? Great. Celebrate your victory. If you didn't, take time to evaluate and learn where you got off track. Critical to this is understanding what is working

and what is not. Occasionally you may need to build a new plan with corrections and new goals.

- **Importance and Confidence.**
  On a scale of 1 to 10, where 10 is extremely important, make sure you are at a 9 or 10. Recognize that in terms of confidence, on a scale of 1 to 10 where 10 is extremely confident, you *can* be at a 1 or a 2, because your confidence will grow as you take steps toward your goal. High importance, a willingness to learn, and a willingness to change will allow you to build confidence along your journey.

- **Know What Works.**
  If you have a goal of weight loss and you are female, 60%–80% of your success will lie in your nutritional plan. If you are male, because of higher testosterone levels, your success can be reached with 60%–80% exercise. Male or female, and for long-term health and success, both nutrition and exercise are important but when you have to prioritize your time or efforts, choose accordingly.

Dream Like a Child

Imagine sitting on Santa's lap and being asked, "What do you want for Christmas?"

A child typically replies without thought: a doll or action figure—because what kid did not want one of those? They ask for a new bike or the last three really cool toys they saw on television. Children are naturally curious and live delightfully in discovery. With every new store they go to, they add to their wish list and leave with an update for Santa.

You have a childlike spirit within you that has those same instincts, emotions, and responses. The difference is that as an adult, you have learned to respond in a more socially acceptable manner. If asked what you want most in life, you may say world peace, or "Nothing. I don't need anything." But the benefit of being an adult is still being able to reply as a child who is in touch with their inner needs. A child who knows their truth. You can ask for the exact things that would make you happier, create ease, and allow you to live a more inspired life.

As a self-reflecting adult thinking about the response of a child, we see that children typically ask for the following kinds of things:

- to do better in school (work)
- to have nicer things (physical possessions)
- to not go to bed hungry (or have more resources)
- to have Mommy and Daddy not fight so much (loving relationships)
- to spend more time with their parents (people they love).

Children see the Universe as Santa's lap. They feel that this is their big chance to get it right, find their truth, be more content, happy, and fulfilled. To make better choices and ultimately make their dreams come true.

Now, this simple four-word question becomes huge. But it's no longer so much of "What do I want?" as it is "What are my dreams?" Asked this way, the answer now deserves a more deliberate response.

What would fulfill me? What will make me happiest? What will fulfill my passions? What would I love? What is best for me? These are all great questions that require a truth that bubbles out of your heart and overflows onto others, brightening everyone's path in the process.

Answer these questions without restrictions, such as, "It's too costly," or "I don't have time." If time and money were no object, what would I want?

Let's look deeper. What would serve you and the world around you? What do you love? What are you passionate about? What can you naturally do well, understand easily or learn to do well? What will benefit the world and truly make a difference?

Start by seeing yourself as grand and worthy, as the Universe sees you, as God sees you. And dream big.

Now that you understand the question, ask yourself again, "What do I want?" Define your inner bliss. Follow your dreams and declare what you really, really want. And then, go build it.

Measure of Success

I love the chunking of time—decades, years, seasons or quarters, months, weeks, days, hours, minutes, seconds—and how it helps to break down goals into more manageable segments. At any given point you have the opportunity to check-in and evaluate how far you've come, and whether you need to adjust to continue on your path to success.

Success is often measured by comparison and competition. It's easy to judge yourself and your performance based on how others around you are doing. But success simply means that at the end of the day, as you look in the mirror, you do so with confidence and humility, knowing that you did your best in comparison to your own ability.

It's OK to Fail

It's ok to fail. In fact, failure is a very important part of any journey. It teaches you what your weaknesses and liabilities are. It tells you what you must learn to have the success you want. It tells you who you are required to be in order to reach the goals you have for yourself.

In cycling with riders who are more advanced than you, you may get dropped (you can't keep up with a group of riders) and fall behind the group. Yes, it sucks. You may even cry. I have. But it happens to us all at one point or another. We all end up riding with someone better than us sooner or later, and chances are, when this happens, we got dropped and then swore to get better. After you get dropped, you work harder than you ever have before. You push yourself a little bit more in those final moments.

In Bikram yoga, you learn to stretch to your maximum point of flexibility (which some might call failure), knowing next time, your body will remember the point at which you left off and continue to improve.

In the gym, they call it "going to failure," and it is a good thing; it's the point where the most growth happens in the muscles. It's called failing forward.

Most would consider quarterback Peyton Manning's rookie season a loss or failure. His team went 3–13. He went on to appear in four Super Bowls, winning two.

Michael Jordan didn't make the cut to play for his high school varsity basketball team. He is one of the greatest basketball players of all time.

Boxing champion Muhammad Ali wasn't a natural fighter and in his early boxing days, was considered a failure by experts.

Baseball legend Babe Ruth holds the record for the most strikeouts and the third-highest home run record.

Regardless of how you look at it, failure is a part of life and part of success.

Internal Motivation

As a wellness consultant, I post a lot of tips, before and after photos, and inspiration / motivation on social media. I do weekly coaching calls, send texts, and guide people along a path. I point people toward the best nutrition on the planet and systems that truly work if you work them. The reality is, change doesn't come from me or some version of external inspiration. Change and success come from within. You must be internally motivated. It happens when you are ready. Change and transformation happen when:

- you are sick and tired of being stuck and want to improve your body, health, or life;
- you realize that there are people in your life that deserve to experience you at your best;
- there are adventures in life that you demand to experience;

- you decide that you want to feel amazing in your body and your life;
- you are really, truly ready to accept responsibility for your own success and failure;
- you declare you will no longer make excuses, you will take off your victim hat, and you will step forward boldly and courageously into your destiny.

The world needs you and you need you to be at your best, living a life of passion and purpose, with fire in your belly, peace in your soul, and love in your heart. A little bit of laughter goes a long way too.

Start with Why

After you decide what you want, the next step to making any healthy lifestyle stick is to know **why** you are making changes toward better health. This will help you stay focused.

When I met my best friend and now husband, we made a promise to each other: to be as healthy as we possibly could be, every single day, for the rest of our lives. I'm counting on him to keep his promise. He's counting on me to keep mine.

That is my "why." That is what motivates me to live a healthy lifestyle every single day to the best of my ability.

Every single one of you has someone or something in your life that is counting on you. It may be your partner, best friend, child, parent, four-legged friend, passion, mission, ministry, or faith.

What is it for you? What is your top priority? What is the thing that would cause you to move heaven and earth to protect it and keep it sacred? The thing that would cause you to act? To change? To rise? To come back strong?

Do you know?

Because if you do, it will make all the difference with your decisions. It will be what drives you to seek balance and wellness and live your best life toward success and happiness.

In a previous section, I wrote that it's important to know what healthy means to you personally. It's just as important—if not more so—to know why you want to live a healthy lifestyle. To uncover this, ask yourself:

- How do you want to feel?
- Who in your life is counting on you to be healthy?
- What family or personal history are you looking to change?

Perhaps you
- want to embrace your inner athlete and compete in your first 5k, marathon, or fitness competition;

- want to feel good in your body;
- want to rock any outfit you put on;
- are the caretaker of a partner, parent, child, or four-legged friend who is counting on and depending on you;
- had a health scare and you're partnering with your medical support team to avoid medication or surgery;
- want to look and feel your best for your wedding, reunion, vacation, or another upcoming event;
- haven't been feeling well, so you are eliminating sugar / dairy / wheat / caffeine to see if it makes a difference.

Knowing why you want to make a healthy change will keep you focused and motivated toward your goals. Having a clear vision of why you want to live a healthy lifestyle will help you choose between what you want now and what you want most. Whatever your reason, own it and embrace it. It will be the driving force that keeps you going even during the times when you want to quit.

Share Your Why

Once you have figured out the reason why you want to live a healthy lifestyle, it's helpful to share that with your support system. You may be tempted to keep your lifestyle changes to yourself. There could be many reasons, such as you are

- independent and want to do this on your own;
- afraid it might not work or you won't stick to it;
- concerned that your relationships will suffer.

A key aspect of your success will lie in the accountability that comes from sharing your decision with your community: your close family, friends, and co-workers—especially those people you surround yourself with.

Cookouts, vacations, reunions, or other social occasions where you will be eating as a group are all events where you will want to tell family and friends your why. Call people ahead of time and let them know some of the changes they can expect, such as that you will

- skip cocktails
- pass on dessert
- seek out extra vegetables and lean meats (and skip the pasta or heavy casseroles)
- take walks after meals

Let them know that it's not easy sticking to your plan, and you'd appreciate their support while you create a healthier lifestyle. Reassure them that your choice of certain foods is personal and not a reflection on them.

Wanting or Willing?

Your why has to be strong. It has to be personal to you and on a scale of 1 to 10 in terms of importance, it has to bring you to at least an 8. When it comes to change, the reality of your success lies in the difference between wanting something to be different and being willing to do whatever it takes to make it happen.

- Wanting keeps you in limbo. Willing takes action and moves you forward.
- Wanting keeps you in "try" mode. Willing puts you in "do" mode.
- Wanting is enslaving. Willing is empowering.
- Wanting results in self-sabotage and failure. Willing results in success, whatever it takes.
- Wanting is indefinite. Willing is definite.

For example:
- You can want to lose weight and never release a pound.
- You can want six-pack abs, and never see them revealed.
- You can want a new job, and find yourself stuck in the same position year after year.
- You can want to get out of debt, and yet sink further and further behind every month.
- You can want to give up caffeine / sugar / alcohol, and yet day after day find yourself a victim to the same habits, cravings, and addictions.
- You can want better relationships and yet never find love or a best friend or always feel lonely.
- You can want to go to Australia, Paris, or Bali, and never leave the comfort of your hometown.

After wanting change day after day, week after week, month after month, year after year, and not seeing change, you will either give up or beat yourself up. Self-love and grace go out the door and you doubt yourself, thinking you simply aren't capable of change.

Today, draw a line in the sand and say: "It's not that I can't do it, it's that up until now, I haven't been willing to commit to doing it. I haven't made a firm decision to do whatever it takes and change whatever is in the way that keeps me from reaching my goal."

Wait.

Say that first part again: *"It's not that I can't do it, it's that up until now, I haven't been willing to commit to doing it."*

Feel that. Let that really sink in. Realize that in this present moment, you can re-evaluate. Ask yourself: Is this something I really want right now in my life, or is it an old dream or goal or someone else's desire for me to change?

If the answer is no, then release it. Let it go. Stop beating yourself up for something you don't truly want.

If the answer is yes, then ask yourself: Am I willing to do what it takes to achieve it?

If the answer is no, WOW! That is powerful. Let yourself off the hook. It may not be the right time, or if you are not willing, it may not truly be what you want. You can always decide to come back to it at a later date. For now, let it go and spend your time focusing on more productive things you truly care about.

If the answer is yes, then take action right now. Send a text or email, make a call, set an appointment with a nutritionist, coach, banker, mentor, prospect, or lawyer to begin the process. Do one thing right now, no matter how small, to solidify what you are saying yes to.

There is a window of willingness right now. It's not later, tomorrow, Monday or next week. It's right now in this present moment where, if you take action, you will solidify your commitment and start the ball rolling toward the change you desire.

It will take passion to do what it takes to change. It will take dedication to move beyond want and to step into willing. Remember, change can be uncomfortable, and discomfort can feel like pain. It is hard to focus on changing when you are focused on discomfort and pain. There is a part of your brain instinctively that wants to protect you from that pain. You may sabotage your efforts by doing things that take you out of that discomfort and lead you away from actions that you must take in order to change.

But change you must. And you, my dear, are worth it.

YOUR TURN

What does healthy mean to you?

_____

_____

What area of your health would you like to improve?

_____

_____

Is there something you've failed at in your life? Did you give up or keep going till you mastered it or at least, felt more comfortable doing it? Explain.

_____

_____

_____

Why do you want to be healthy?

_____

_____

Who in your life is counting on you to be healthy?

_____

List three people with whom you will share your "why" before the end of the week:

_____

_____

_____

Transform

CHAPTER 2

Sabotage

AS YOU WORK TOWARD creating more consistency in your healthy lifestyle, there will inevitably be setbacks, challenges, and obstacles that rear their ugly head. Having advanced knowledge on how to overcome them provides confidence that you will succeed.

Peaks and Valleys

Along the journey toward success, there are always distractions, both good and bad. Life throws curve balls. There are ups and downs, peaks and valleys. Stuff happens. Stay committed anyway.

We've all been there before. We decide to make changes, eat better, get to the gym, and something happens. We get sick, or our day gets so busy we miss our workout, or a meeting gets scheduled during lunch and all of a sudden we're starving and the only option is the vending machine or fast-food restaurant on the corner. And just like that, our healthy lifestyle is derailed. Again.

The dog dies. Your lover / partner leaves you. You undergo surgery. You get the flu, or worse, are diagnosed with an illness. A global pandemic hits and you are forced into retirement. Your partner gets laid off. The gyms close. You are lucky enough to work from home but you are also responsible for keeping your kids on task with their remote learning.

And then there are the GOOD distractions. You move. Fall in love. Find a church home. Get married. Change jobs. Win a sports competition or fitness challenge. Buy a new car. Go on a missions trip.

Good or bad, distractions still have the potential to derail us from the things we set out to do. Success will come when you embrace the mindset that no matter what comes, come hell or high water, you will finish what you start. You will offer yourself patience and grace through the natural ebb and flow of success.

My road to finalist in the sixteen-week challenges was not a straight line to success. In fact, it was filled with peaks and valleys. There were setbacks, obstacles, and seasons where it was easier to make excuses than push on toward success.

In 2014, I signed up for the sixteen-week challenge. I got super focused. I was all in. I counted down the weeks and days on my calendar. I asked my trainer—my husband—for help. I felt amazing. I was in the best shape of my life. I was confident I was going to be a finalist. *Peak*.

I waited. And waited. Then watched as, one by one, all five finalists were announced. I was devastated. *Valley*.

Then, the call came in: I was an honorable mention. *Peak*.

During my next challenge, an unexpected surgery sent me into sudden surgical menopause. Most people associate menopause with hot flashes. No big deal. My experience was different. For the next 18 months, my body, mind, and emotions tanked. I couldn't sleep. I couldn't focus. I had no drive, passion, or purpose. Despite doing everything I had done in the past, I gained weight. I went to the doctors looking for answers. They told me to adjust my perspective; this was all part of aging. I lost hope. *Valley*.

I felt old beyond my years and before my time. I lost my sense of vitality and wellbeing. *Valley*.

Rock bottom came during a conversation with my husband when I was feeling my worst. It felt like he had pulled back; like HE had disappeared. To which he replied, "What? Are you kidding me? Lori, YOU disappeared."

That scared me. *Valley*.

And, it woke me up.

In the valley, we grow and change. We find our grit.

A few weeks later, a friend was announced as a 2017 finalist. We recommitted to the challenge and during those sixteen weeks, Jim became a finalist (and then runner-up). Jim's body responded quicker than mine. Now he was on the mountain peak, and I was still climbing.

But you know what? The best view comes after the hardest climb. I have built my support team and surrounded myself with other finalists, a corporate team, and a Facebook group filled with members who are climbing their mountains and facing their valleys. Each of them has cheered me on. "Don't give up. Keep going. You can do this."

And, I believe them.

The community of support is the mountain peak. Humans long for love and connection. The community inspired me to find my confidence, my smile, and my six-pack abs.

Regardless of where you are, the peak or the valley, you can continue to rise. You can continue to climb each and every mountain before you.

Regardless of where you are, you can come back strong. And always, enjoy the journey.

Obstacles to a Healthy Lifestyle and How to Overcome Them

I'm too tired to work out. Eating healthy is too expensive. I'm so busy, I don't have time to cook my own meals. I don't know where to begin. I'll start on Monday.

If you're like most people, you've probably used or heard one of these excuses when faced with a goal to eat better and / or exercise more. And you probably had trouble sticking to your healthy lifestyle. There are many common obstacles you may come up against as you start to make changes. However, a bit of planning, knowledge, and support can move you past them and toward a healthy lifestyle. Below are some of the most common obstacles, along with tips to overcome them.

I don't have time

Eating healthy and exercising requires time. With so much to do and so little time to do it, things can easily slip through the cracks. This is one area where multitasking can come in handy. Weaving relationships into an active lifestyle allows you to nurture two priorities in one time slot (more on this in chapter 3).

Typically, relationships are built and maintained by gathering around food and alcohol.

Instead, consider this:
- Date nights can become date rides where you and your partner get out on your bicycles.
- Family day can include a 5k run / walk for charity, miniature golf, or a scavenger hunt.
- Friendships can be centered around a hike, snowshoeing, or fitness class.
- Your spiritual relationship can combine prayer and meditation with a walk in nature.

I don't have any support

In fact, it feels like the people in your life are sabotaging your efforts. You start a new diet and your co-worker shows up with bagels, brownies, or birthday cake. You are disciplined all week and your sister calls to invite you out for ice cream or happy hour. You start a cleanse and your partner decides to make your favorite meal of spaghetti and meatballs and homemade garlic cheesy bread. Those closest to you can be your biggest support or they can sabotage your efforts without even knowing it.

As we discussed in chapter one, the best thing you can do to gain support is to tell the people you interact with most often with the reason *why* you are making changes toward a healthier lifestyle. When you tell people why you want to be healthy, they are more prepared to rally around you and even hold you accountable. Ask them for suggestions of activities they would enjoy with you that don't center on food. We'll cover this more in chapter three.

I just want to do this on my own

Sometimes, the opposite happens: you are not looking for support. You want to keep your healthy lifestyle to yourself until people notice your results. This is a surefire way to fail. Even if you have strong willpower and self-discipline, it's hard to make changes on your own without support and accountability. You weren't meant to do life alone. Friends and family can be your biggest supporters and accountability partners if you let them. They will cheer for you over victories and encourage you when you feel like giving up. Again, as we discussed in chapter one, the key is communication. Tell your close circle of friends and family why you are doing this and ask for their help. They may help with meal planning or finding alternative activities. They may even join you. At the very least, they will no longer unknowingly sabotage you.

I'm too tired

Sometimes the obstacle in your way is fatigue. Life gets so busy, you start to skip your workouts. If you haven't planned ahead, you are too tired to cook and it's easy to order a pizza or other quick takeout meal. While these foods aren't necessarily right or wrong, they do contain more salt, sugar, and fat than the food you cook at home. Lack of exercise and the wrong foods can add to your fatigue.

This obstacle requires a closer look at the source of your fatigue. Are you sleeping at night? Is your calendar too full? Are you rising early and staying up late? Are you on medications that might be causing drowsiness? How much caffeine is in your system? Is something you are eating causing your tiredness (think turkey at Thanksgiving)? When was the last time you took a vacation (burnout)?

Sleep and nutrition are so underestimated when it comes to energy and exhaustion. Ask yourself: Can I go to bed early or sleep late? Can I take a nap? Can I cut back on caffeine? What are my bedtime routines for winding down and relaxing? Next, take a look at your nutrition. Home cooking offers less salt, sugar, and harmful additives and can save you time and effort by providing leftovers for a future meal. As sleep and nutrition improve, you'll find you feel less tired for your workouts, giving you more energy.

I'm too stressed

Stress shows up in our life on a daily basis. It comes from major life events such as the death of a loved one, marriage, divorce, job promotion, or job loss as well as the cumulative build-up of everyday frustrations from living your life. You work hard, it's important that you make time to play and rest, too.

Monitor your days so you don't burn the candle at both ends. Learn to say no to things that don't align with your priorities. Guard your calendar as if your life depended on it. Your health does. Finally, find a way to bring more balance to your life with meditation, walks in nature, play, and just plain FUN.

It's too boring

If a healthy lifestyle is not fun for you, you just might be doing it wrong. Exercise can involve something you love, whether that's cycling, skiing, yoga, volleyball, or kayaking. Don't know what it is you enjoy? What did you love to do as a child? Do that.

Healthy meals at home can also be fun with family and friends. Buffet style works great for an all-inclusive meal where guests can make and build their own. You could do grain or salad bowls, tacos, shish-kabobs, or soups and stews. They all start with a vegetable base and participants can add their choice of protein, potatoes, rice, beans, lentils, or quinoa. Even burgers, fries, and pizza can be made with less fat, salt, and dairy and more vegetables, herbs, and spices. An air-fryer can be your best friend as an alternate way to cook your favorite foods that are traditionally fried.

Healthy food doesn't taste as good

Do you remember your first cup of coffee? How about your first drink of alcohol? Did you love it? Chances are you had to acquire a taste for it over time. Your taste buds get accustomed to what you eat. If you drink coffee or eat sugar and salt daily, that's your routine and that's what your taste buds are used to. You can just as easily train your palate—and your mind—to like the taste of healthy food. And it doesn't have to be bland or boring. There are some amazing herbs and seasonings that can tantalize your taste buds.

I'm too social

Some jobs require networking and social events that revolve around food. It may be dinner with clients or a mixer after work. Maneuvering this obstacle requires planning, preparation, and decision-making. Decide ahead of time to skip alcohol, appetizers, or dessert. Review the menu before you arrive at the restaurant and make a plan to choose the healthiest option ahead of time when you are not hungry or listening to what everyone else is choosing. For the networking events, eat a healthy meal in advance and ask for water with a lime or cherry while you mingle.

I don't know where to start

It can be overwhelming to start something new. Maybe you assume you have to go from couch potato to CrossFit competitor overnight. That is why so many New Year's resolutions fail by February. You bite off more than you can chew, try to change everything all at once, and fizzle out before making progress.

The key is to start small. Maybe for you, it's five minutes of daily walking. Or taking one lunch hour to exercise each week. You could cut back on caffeine, sugar, or sodium. You could add in a weekly family dinner where you make a healthier version of your favorite meal. Small actions done with consistency are the key to starting and maintaining a healthier lifestyle.

It's too expensive

Have you ever added up what you spend on food, snacks, supplements, and drinks on a daily basis? It can be a real eye-opener. Take the next two weeks and write everything you buy and consume. Include groceries, coffee, energy drinks, sports supplements, vending machine snacks, even popcorn at the movies. Calculate what you are spending on a daily basis. Then ask yourself, "Are my purchases supporting my desire for a healthier lifestyle?" Healthier foods may be more expensive, but if they provide you with better nutrients, you'll find you have more energy and fewer cravings for junk food. You may even experience greater productivity in your work and less time off due to illness.

Gym memberships can be expensive, but exercise and moving your body don't require a gym. You can walk, run, bike, ski, swim, or snowshoe with minimal equipment. A TRX® or Total Gym® are great tools you can buy one time and reap the benefits long term. YouTube can help you with tips on bodyweight exercises that you can do anywhere, such as pull-ups, pushups, situps, squats, and lunges. There are plenty of free yoga offerings as well. If you are completely lost or a beginner, find a local personal trainer. Ask if they have a special offer where they show you how to get started and then give you exercises to continue with on your own.

Procrastination

I'll wait till Monday. Or the New Year. Or when I'm older. The best time to make changes toward a healthier lifestyle is now. Someone in your life is counting on you, whether it's your partner, child, parent, co-worker, or best friend (including the four-legged ones). Maybe, it's YOU counting on you. You desire to live your best, healthiest life with freedom in your body, your clothes, and your life.

You don't have to wait. You can start today, this very moment, to make small, consistent changes toward a healthier lifestyle. Grab a glass of water and hydrate your cells. Take a few minutes to stretch or get outside for a walk. Even five minutes can make a difference. Set the alarm for 30 minutes earlier and start tomorrow with movement and meditation. Remember, a healthy lifestyle is lived with small actions done consistently over time.

Don't be afraid to ask for help. Talk to other people and be open to suggestions. Think of someone you admire and ask them how they got to where they are and how they maintain their status. People love to share their success.

Triggers

While you want to gain support from your family and friends and avoid common obstacles and excuses, you also need to be aware of other factors and triggers that can sabotage your goals, especially when it comes to eating healthy.

To understand food triggers, it helps to understand the four key chemicals that make you feel wonderful and can help you to accomplish your goals. They include serotonin, dopamine, endorphins, and oxytocin.

Serotonin is a hormone that helps to stabilize your mood, supporting feelings of wellbeing and happiness.[1] You can't get serotonin directly from food, but you can get tryptophan, an amino acid that is converted to serotonin in your brain. You can increase serotonin levels through exercise, bright lights, supplements, or massage.

Dopamine[2] is a feel-good neurotransmitter that is associated with happiness. It's a chemical that ferries information between neurons. The brain releases it when we eat food that we crave or during sex, contributing to feelings of pleasure and satisfaction as part of the reward system. To increase dopamine, add more protein to your diet and less saturated fats, consume probiotics, exercise, get good quality and quantity sleep, listen to music, meditate, and spend time in the sun.

When endorphins[3] are released they can help relieve pain, reduce stress, and may cause a euphoric feeling. They are released during exercise, acupuncture, massage, meditation, aromatherapy, and sex. They can also be released by drinking wine or eating dark chocolate, laughing, practicing random acts of kindness, performing music, or taking a hot bath.

Oxytocin[4] is a hormone and a neurotransmitter that is involved in childbirth and breastfeeding. It is also associated with empathy, trust, sex, and relationship-building. It is sometimes referred to as the love hormone because levels of oxytocin increase during hugging and orgasm. Hugging, kissing, cuddling, and sexual intimacy can all trigger oxytocin production, which can strengthen bonds between adults. Other ways to produce oxytocin include listening to or making music, having sex, giving or receiving a massage, having sex, telling someone you care about them, hanging out with friends, having sex, meditating, actively listening to a friend, cooking and eating with someone you care about, having sex, doing something nice for someone, or petting your animals. Oh, and did I mention having sex?

These chemicals are required for mental stability and strength, so choose ways to make and increase them so they contribute to accomplishing your goals.

Here are some triggers that can sabotage your goals when it comes to eating healthy.

Chemical imbalances

Certain foods trigger the release of dopamine, a feel-good neurotransmitter in the brain. Caffeine, salt, sugar, fats (fried or fatty foods), alcohol, MSG, and artificial sweeteners are all added to food with the goal of increasing dopamine, which causes an internal chemical reward that increases the likelihood that eating those foods will become habitual. This feel-good dopamine reward encourages you to eat more unhealthy foods. This is a built-in addictive mechanism that keeps you craving certain foods. In addition, these foods are often grown or prepared in a manner that makes them abundant, cheap, and easily accessible, but they are typically not foods that preserve, secure or strengthen your health.

Addictive chemicals in our food

Food manufacturers are well aware of this addictive reaction and will add these addictive chemicals to our food to increase repeat purchases of their products. The good news is that as you decrease caffeine, salt, sugar, fats (fried or fatty foods), alcohol, MSG, and artificial sweeteners from your diet, you'll begin to crave them less and break your habit or addiction to them.

A general rule is to beware of foods that break down your self-discipline and control; those foods where you can't eat just one, or they leave you craving more of other things.

Food sensitivities

In addition to these dopamine-enhancing additives are foods that can cause sensitivities and inflammation, which will block weight loss for you personally. These sensitivities are individualized in that they may affect you but not affect others. They may even be considered healthy foods. Common foods that cause inflammation and / or sensitivities include soy, eggs, fish, shellfish, tree nuts, peanuts, gluten, or whey protein.

Sometimes the scale is the only indicator that you are sensitive to a food or a food is causing inflammation. If the scale continues to go up or if it jumps up and down from day to day, even though you feel you are doing everything right consistently to maintain or release weight, you may want to consider if you are reacting to something you eat every day.

Other times your body gives you clues. For years I ate eggs and whey protein daily, thinking I was eating healthy. But I had a case of chronic constipation and idiopathic hives that said differently. Nothing showed up as an allergy in any of the tests my doctors did. However, once I took an at-home food sensitivity test, I discovered that my body was having an immune response to these two foods. I eliminated both from my diet and both the hives and constipation resolved.

Your emotions

You may also have emotional triggers that cause you to binge eat or eat unhealthy foods. When your brain is too active, such as when you are anxious or tense, you can use food to numb yourself in an effort to slow down brain waves to make yourself more comfortable. On the other hand, if your brain is underactive and you feel bored or sad, food can be used to stimulate your brain waves to make you more comfortable. Sometimes, food helps you to feel full when your life feels empty.

I eat when I'm bored, stressed, and anxious. I also eat when I'm not doing what I want to do or when I'm procrastinating. Discontent is my worst instigator for overeating. On the other hand, when I'm writing, gardening, or riding my bike, I am rarely thinking about food.

Simple awareness of when and why you are eating can help resolve your emotional eating. If you feel hungry, start by drinking a glass of water and wait twenty minutes. You may be confusing thirst and hunger. During your wait time, check-in with your emotions to assess whether you are truly physically hungry, or if you are trying to suppress feelings of boredom, sadness, anxiety, or tension. If you start to notice that you eat when you are emotional, then try to resolve that emotion without relying on food. If you are bored, find something to keep you busy and take your mind off of food. Go for a walk, answer email, or clean out a junk drawer. If you are sad or anxious, consider talking to a friend or therapist. If you eat when you are tense, consider stress-reducing tools such as yoga, meditation, or deep breathing.

Irregular eating or not having a plan

Being overly hungry can also serve as a trigger to binge eat. If you eat at irregular times or skip meals, you may try to satisfy your feelings of being hungry with more calories than are necessary. Then, as a result of eating too many calories, you try to make up for the binge by being overly strict with your diet. This is a cycle that can be hard to break.

Eating smaller meals at regular intervals such as every few hours will help keep you satiated. Split your lunch into two meals and add in a mid-morning and mid-afternoon snack. Make sure your meals and snacks have a balance of low glycemic carbohydrates, lean protein, and essential fatty acids. This will help you avoid blood sugar drops and spikes that trigger binge eating or impulse eating of foods not on our plan.

Body image issues

In today's social media-driven world, there is an unhealthy amount of pressure to have the perfect body. While this used to be mainly a female issue, avoiding the "dad bod" in recent years has added this pressure to men as well. This pressure combined with low self-esteem can cause excessive frustration and trigger binge eating.

In your quest to live a healthy lifestyle, remember that while it is good to have health and fitness goals and standards, your journey is also about finding inner peace and happiness, not simply a physical result. Maintaining this perspective will allow your body image issues to be more manageable. In extreme cases, speaking with a counselor or psychiatrist may be needed. Asking for help is not a weakness; it is a strength and can often help move you forward faster than if you try to do it alone.

Combination of factors

Sometimes, it is a combination of factors that can trigger binge eating. For example, a difficult work schedule may prevent you from keeping a healthy eating schedule, causing you to binge eat, followed by the feeling of depression.

Other stuff

You have beliefs that either serve you in leading a healthy lifestyle or that don't. If you are willing to change those beliefs that are getting in the way of your dreams, goals, success, or happiness, then habits and rules in chapter four will help you recreate a mindset that supports rather than sabotages you.

Food Cravings

Pizza. Chocolate. Gummy bears. Sugar. Salt. Bolivian food. These were some of the answers I received when I asked around on social media about the obstacles people struggle with most when it comes to living a healthy lifestyle. And it's not just what you eat, but how much you eat that can be an obstacle.

I am no stranger to food cravings or addictions. Pizza and wine, burgers and beer, cookies, brownies, ice cream...don't get me started, or I literally will not stop. While I may have been able to get away with eating a pint of Ben and Jerry's for dinner in my teens and twenties, with every added decade I require a little more discipline. Add in surgical menopause, and my eating requires even stricter and more consistent nutritional guidelines.

What I have found is that it is easy to get into a habit of rewarding myself with these foods I crave. And, it takes consistency over time to create new healthy habits (coming up in chapter four) while breaking the old ones.

A healthy lifestyle is all about feeling your best. But in some cases, it is also a matter of life and death. If you have had (or someone in your family history has had) a cardiological or an oncological complication, if you have diabetes, or if you suffer from illness or disease, food makes all the difference in the quantity and quality of your life. Knowing why you want to be healthy (as discussed in chapter one) and building a support network (coming up in chapter three) is crucial to your success and longevity.

Rewards and Cheat Meals

You've been good all week and you think, just one cookie. One beer. A burger. The truth is, eating crappy food is not a reward. It's a punishment.

Throughout the diet and fitness world is the idea of building in a cheat meal at regular intervals. A cheat meal is a preplanned exception to your healthy lifestyle that you decide to make ahead of time. This exception or cheat meal will set you back on your way to your building ironclad habits. It will not propel you toward building ironclad habits. And unfortunately, a cheat meal often turns into a cheat day, a cheat weekend, or an ongoing habit of daily cheats that derail you from your goals.

You are not a dog. You don't need to reward or treat yourself with "cheat" food for being good for staying on your diet or healthy lifestyle plan for a few days. On the contrary, eating crappy food punishes you and your health in the long run. It slows down your progress toward your goals. You are compromising your long-term health for short-term pleasure, and compromise destroys rather than builds great habits.

By continuing to build in cheat meals with unhealthy foods, you keep yourself in a bad habit. You also will continue to crave and desire these foods. While you are first implementing your healthier habits, you need to distance yourself from cheat meals and food rewards. It's not to say you will never enjoy foods with sugar, salt, or even alcohol ever again. It just means you are choosing to eat in a way that is consistent with your goals. Give up the "I have been good all week so I deserve" mentality.

What you deserve is to feel good in your body, your clothes, and your health. You deserve to relax, exercise, and eat well. Your body is a temple. Fuel it. Explore alternative ways to reward yourself such as a massage, new outfit, or trip to visit friends or family. These make a great goal and reward after a successful month of healthy living.

Holiday Binging

As a child, the holidays were bookmarked with two dates: December 13th, my sister's birthday, was the date we traditionally set up our Christmas tree, and January 1st, the day we took it down. We enjoyed three weeks of festivity, food, family, and cheer.

These days, the holiday season has been extended to start as early as Halloween and carry through to New Year's, Valentine's, St. Patrick's Day, or even Easter! We are bombarded in stores, on TV, social media, email, and the radio. I'd like to believe that this extension is filled with joy, peace, and love, yet I know that the reality is it can be a time of stress and overeating.

As early as Halloween we begin to fill our bodies with foods that were meant for a day—hence the term holi-day, not holi-week or holi-month.

We feel the effects physically, mentally, and emotionally. We spend money we don't have, and desperately hope for a tax refund to pay off our credit card. The merging of families can create a brilliant juggling act of scheduling dates and holiday get-togethers. Add in friends, work, religious services, and our schedule overflows. Hopefully with abundance, but often, overwhelm.

All these factors can make us feel negative emotions which lead us to feel "less than" or broken. How do we stay healthy during this season? How do we stay whole? How do we spread joy, love, hope, and peace to everyone we encounter, and most importantly, to ourselves?

Staying whole for the holidays is a delicate balance of loving others and ourselves.

Consider this: the traditional holiday dinner packs an average of 3,000 calories.[5] The recommended daily caloric intake for women ranges from 1,400 to 2,000, putting *one holiday meal* at approximately a third more than a full day's requirement.

Add to that the busyness around the holiday, skipped workouts, stress, and extra socializing, and we can feel out of sorts by the time the holiday is over.

Here are a few tips to keep your holiday healthier and on track with your goals.

- **Plan a post-meal walk or other activity.** Depending on the weather, plan to get outside for a walk or game of family football. Have a fitness instructor in the family? Ask them to do a mid-day "class" to get everyone moving. If you are stuck indoors, a Wii or other game system will get you moving, and if all else fails, turn on some music and dance.
- **Move around and mingle.** Avoid the kitchen or appetizer area where you are tempted to graze.
- **Plan a workout date** with your partner or a friend for the morning before, the day of, and the day after the holiday.
- **Practice portion control.** By keeping your portions small, you can still enjoy your favorite holiday dishes.
- **Fill your plate with protein and veggies first.** Then, for your second round, enjoy smaller portions of the more decadent dishes.
- **Hydrate.** This will keep hunger at bay.
- **Skip it.** Decide what you can live without. Perhaps the appetizers, the alcohol, or the dessert. Each one alone could easily add 1,000 calories to your day.
- Not hosting? **Bring a healthy dish to pass**, like a salad or veggie platter.
- **Eat slowly.** Eating slowly gives your body enough time to realize that you're full.

- **Stay active.** Stick to your workouts, even if you have to shorten them temporarily. Remember to schedule it on your calendar just like any other important engagement.
- **Get quality sleep.** Sleep can become something we sacrifice when the holiday season kicks in. You may stay up late to wrap gifts or clean the house, trying to fit it all in. Or you get up early to get that extra workout in. It is not worth sacrificing your health and emotional wellbeing. Everything in life becomes more difficult without good quality sleep.
- **Reduce stress.** It is common to want a vacation to reduce our stress, but that's not always an option. Incorporate daily activities that help you reduce stress, whether it be yoga, meditation, a walk outside, or even a gratitude journal.
- Finally—**have FUN** during the holiday. Enjoy the traditions and mix in some healthy activities and recipes.

You Drink Too Much

"You drink too much to lose weight."

That was what my friend Kate told me years ago. Ouch. Really? At the time I didn't think so. Wine has so many benefits, the least of all the calming effect, which can lower stress. However, if weight loss is the goal, I encourage you to do a 30-day alcohol fast. If you drink daily, the first few days may be tough, but what I have found is that in the long run, my head is clearer, my energy is higher, and the weight comes off quicker.

Consider this: One glass of your favorite alcoholic drink can shut your metabolism down for 36 hours. So picture this: You start your weekend early with a drink on Thursday. Then, of course, wine with dinner Friday and Saturday. Sunday you have a beer at the barbecue. Monday you go back to your stricter healthy lifestyle and no alcohol. Tuesday you're sticking to it. And by Wednesday your metabolism kicks in and you enter weight loss mode. Then, Thursday, you are back to your weekend cycle and all your weight loss goals go out the window.

You may be eating a generally healthy diet, but if you're not seeing results it may be because of your alcohol intake. Drinking alcohol and weight loss don't go well together because alcohol can change the way your body burns fat. When you drink, your body is more focused on breaking down alcohol rather than burning fat.

If you need more of a deterrent, consider that drinking too much on a single occasion or over time can take a serious toll on your health. Here's how alcohol can affect your body:

- **Brain:** Alcohol interferes with the brain's communication pathways and can affect the way the brain looks and works.

These disruptions can change mood and behavior, and make it harder to think clearly and move with coordination.

- **Heart:** Drinking a lot over a long time or too much on a single occasion can damage the heart.
- **Liver:** Heavy drinking takes a toll on the liver, and can lead to a variety of problems and liver inflammations.
- **Pancreas:** Alcohol causes the pancreas to produce toxic substances that can eventually lead to pancreatitis, a dangerous inflammation and swelling of the blood vessels in the pancreas that prevents proper digestion.
- **Cancer:** Based on extensive reviews of research studies, there is a strong scientific consensus of an association between alcohol drinking and several types of cancer.
- **Immune system:** Drinking too much can weaken your immune system, making your body a much easier target for disease. Drinking a lot on a single occasion slows your body's ability to ward off infections, even up to 24 hours after getting drunk.

I'm not telling you to never drink a drop of alcohol ever again, I'm just encouraging you to think about what you want now (a glass of wine) versus what you want most (a healthy body and mind).

Wishes, Hopes, Buts, and Fear—What's in Your Way

"I wish I could lose weight. I wish I had more energy. I wish I was in better shape. I wish I didn't feel so old. I wish I had more time."

"But I don't have enough time. But I'm not ready. But I don't have enough money."

Sound familiar? It is possible that these excuses are in the way of your goals, success, and dreams.

Your words are powerful. When the goal is transformation, examine your language to become more aware of what you are speaking into existence. Be careful with sentences that begin with "I hope," "I wish," "But," and "I'm afraid." Even thinking them can make you feel disempowered.

- **The "I Hope" Person:** I hope I can do it. I hope I can make it. I hope I can keep up. I hope I'm fast enough. I hope I'm strong enough. I hope I'm good enough.
- **The "I Wish" Person:** I wish I could lose weight. I wish I could fit in those jeans. I wish I had more energy. I wish I was in better shape. I wish I was faster. I wish I did not feel so old. I wish I had more time. I wish I had the confidence. I wish I had a better job. I wish I had more money.

- **Is there a problem with the size of your BUT?** But I don't have enough time. But I have to wait till after the holiday. But I have to do more research. But I don't know enough yet. But I'm not ready. But I don't have enough money. But I feel like I can't. But I have to lose weight before I start.
- **Are you the "Give in to Fear" Person?** I'm afraid I will fail. I'm afraid I can't. I'm afraid of what people will think. I'm afraid I'm not disciplined enough. I'm afraid I don't know enough. I'm afraid I'll waste money.

"I remember saying once to my husband, Blake, on the eve of my return to Broadway after a 35 years absence, 'You know, I'm really feeling VERY frightened about this' and I began to tear up. He simply replied, 'Darling, did you actually expect to feel anything else?' I remembered—yet again—that fear is a part of life. The trick is to recognize it and then press on anyway. In fact, the REAL TRICK is to stop focusing on oneself and start focusing on others."
~ Julie Andrews, University of Colorado Boulder Commencement Speech, 2013

Perspective plays a huge role in how you embrace your transformation. When you are facing change, you can encounter fear, excitement, or both at the same time. Fear and excitement are interpreted exactly the same in your brain chemistry. The chemicals that are released in your body are the same. It just boils down to how you decide to name it.

To keep things in perspective and stay positive, embrace the following keys to success.

- **Start with a dream:** Focus on your dream with passion. Embrace it as your new reality. If you don't know exactly what your dream is, live in your curiosity. Your dreams won't necessarily be easy, but if they are worth having, they are worth working hard for.
- **Set goals:** Your goals should be written and have a specific completion date. This will keep you on task and focused. You will be able to identify behaviors that move you toward your goals and behaviors that move you away from them.
- **Make a plan:** This is a detailed step-by-step plan of how you will go from where you are now to where you want to be. It has specific dates attached to each step, and these must be measurable and reviewable. You have periodic reviews and these detailed plans are changed to make them more effective, more realistic, and more accomplishable. These are the A, B, C's of a healthy lifestyle.
  - We all have our start point.

- ○ We all have our journey.
- ○ Seek help from an experienced and successful coach. It is invaluable.

- **Now take action:** Put your plan into play with the support of people who have taken or are taking the same journey you have and have common goals, desires, and focus. You are the sum of your five closest influences.
- **You will have bad days. You will make mistakes:** Learn from them. They are your greatest gift. They tell you what is in between you and the success that you want.
- **Remember this:** It's not just about weight loss, more energy, better performance, maintaining health as you age, and funding your passion. It is about who you become in this process. That transformation happens as you take this journey.
- **Acknowledge and embrace the new YOU each step of the journey:** Celebrate each milestone as well as the small victories. Feel proud that you are living a life of balanced wellness.

Something's Off—Spokes

Physical health is only one part of a thriving life. You can eat healthily and exercise regularly, but if you have few friends, hate your job, or live paycheck to paycheck, then you're not thriving, you are striving, surviving, or struggling. Over time, these issues can affect your emotional and physical health.

In my book, *Come Back Strong: Balanced Wellness after Surgical Menopause,* I wrote

> *I see wellness as a balancing act, much like riding a bicycle.*

> *A bicycle s made up of two wheels composed of a tire, inner tube, and the wheel itself. The wheel is composed of an inner hub and outer rim, which are connected by a series of spokes. Bicycle spokes work together to support and evenly distribute the weight of the rider. On its own, a single spoke is easily bent. Put together with its fellow spokes and it supports a great deal of weight without bending. When one spoke does bend or break, all the other spokes take on more of the load. The extra pressure makes every other spoke more vulnerable to failure. In addition, damaged spokes can cause punctures to the wheel or get caught in your frame, causing you to fall. Every single spoke matters.*

In life, just like on a bike, I've learned that it's important to keep my spokes in good working condition, so I can stay balanced and continue moving forward toward a life of wellness. The spokes in my wellness wheel include nutrition, exercise, faith / spirituality, relationships, finances, self-care / self-love, career, nature, prayer and meditation, rest, passions, purpose, play, and more. Together, they support my healthy lifestyle. When one of these areas or spokes is not working, all other areas are vulnerable.

There are times when it feels like all the spokes in your wheels to wellness are in pretty good condition. You are moving forward toward your goals and dreams with a sense of peace. If one spoke is bent or broken, you can focus on repairing it individually.

Other times, it may feel like all your spokes are broken and every single area of your life needs attention. Using the wheels to wellness analogy and knowing the important spokes in your life can help you examine your life and seek solutions to regain your balance.

YOUR TURN

What excuses or obstacles get in the way of you living a healthy lifestyle?

_____

_____

What triggers sabotage you?

_____

_____

What are the top three spokes in your wellness wheel?

_____

_____

_____

How can you incorporate those priorities into your healthy lifestyle?

_____

_____

_____

Transform

CHAPTER 3

Support

IT'S WIDELY UNDERSTOOD THAT social support can help you achieve your health goals, and who better to provide that support than your partner, family, and friends?

Your inner circle can be a source of encouragement, workout buddies, and a sounding board when things get tough. But sometimes, your support systems can inadvertently sabotage your goals.

Maybe your friends push for fast food when you would rather go to a healthier restaurant, or decide to watch a movie when you had agreed to play mini-golf together. Maybe your partner brings home takeout when you were planning to cook a healthy meal yourself. Maybe it's an offhand comment that hurts your confidence. Whatever it might be, it's often a small thing that they don't even realize is affecting you. So how do we address stuff like this in a nice way and get our loved ones to go from sabotage (inadvertent as it may be) to support?

It's time to create a system of support, accountability, and encouragement. Ignore this step and you will negate your efforts and put friends and family in a position to sabotage you instead of support you. Those closest to you can be your biggest support, or they can do the most damage. They can sabotage your efforts without even knowing it.

Sometimes you may need to build a new support group if your current circle does not understand and support your efforts. Your success depends on surrounding yourself with "like-minded" people that will encourage you and hold you accountable to your goals. This doesn't mean you let go of your current friends or kick your family to the curb. But it may mean that you need to set boundaries on those relationships and redefine how you choose to spend time with them.

Find people who inspire you and who you in turn can inspire. This creates a powerful sensation of hope that will propel you through a bad day. Hope renews your strength during a rough patch. Hope brings peace, understanding, and a sense of community. With this, we begin to share a sense of responsibility for each other. We are better together.

Surround Yourself

You are your own person. However, research shows that you will be greatly influenced by the people you surround yourself with. If your desire is to improve in a sport, seek out athletes that are stronger and faster than you or have achieved the success you desire. Don't be afraid to be the slowest or the least experienced. Surrounding yourself with greatness will challenge you to achieve your own greatness.

If your goal is to eat a healthier diet, then be sure to reach out to friends with similar goals. You can also explore social media, Meetup.com, or Eventbrite for groups to join that will offer you the support and encouragement you require. Can't find one in your local community? Start your own at work, church, or the local community center or YMCA.

Be Coachable

As a runner for 24+ years, I loved the independence. I could strap on my shoes and fly solo out the door on my time and at my own pace. That being said, I am the first to admit I was also a very half-assed or half-fast runner.

I started training in the weight room in 2007. I didn't know anything about lifting weights, so I joined a Progressive Resistance Training Class that was offered at the college I worked at. It is so easy for me to be independent and want to do it my own way. But my way can sometimes get me stuck, especially when I'm not learning as fast as I think I should.

In that class and others, I learned to shut up and listen to the instructor. I learned to trust the people that had gone before me and had something to teach me. I learned to be open to listening.

If there's something askew in your life, then change is required and you have to learn to be coachable. When coaches show up in your life, realize that they have done their time. They have sweat equity. Don't argue. Don't question. Give up the need to be right, and instead learn from the experts.

Coaching is a partnership. The coach has the experience that will help you succeed. Your role as the person being coached is to be coachable.

What exactly does that mean? It means you practice some key character traits:

- **Be open:** Be open (willing and able) to listen and truly hear constructive criticism and feedback without getting defensive. You may have to get uncomfortable, but stay engaged, don't disconnect. When you are open to hearing from an outside source or perspective about what is going on, you can reach new levels of development and progress. Get the honest, complete big picture. Invite and appreciate the feedback, and above all else, do not take anything personally.
- **Be committed to change:** We all have areas to improve. We do not have to strive for perfection; we should all strive for excellence. Take responsibility for your life, your future. Step outside your comfort zone and grow.
- **Get in action:** Be willing to get off your butt and take action.
- **Humility:** Be willing to ask for help. Take a hand up (not a handout). "Humility requires a change of heart rather than a change of mind" (August Turak). Embrace the ideas and assistance of others.
- **Willingness to surrender control:** It is human nature to wait for a crisis or hit rock bottom before we change. The reality is that the reason we hit rock bottom is because of our unwillingness to give up control. Doing it our way is what got us into the situation we need that requires coaching. Be willing to get out of your own way, and surrender. The only way you will see results and be successful is to give up control and trust your coach.
- **Faith:** Hindsight is 20 / 20. It may take time for you to see the benefits of change. Things sometimes get worse before they get better. Trust the process. Stay the course. Each day you can look back and say, "I'm not where I want to be but I'm further along than I used to be."
- **Know thyself:** Develop awareness about yourself. Reflect on your behavior and how it impacts the future you as well as other people.

Stronger Together

In the weight room, people came and went and came back again. During that season in my life and in my training, I was grateful for the people that worked out with me, coached me, encouraged me, pushed me, and believed in me. There were days where I had to borrow from their beliefs. It always paid off. The accountability and support kept me excited, motivated, and growing stronger than I could on my own.

I've seen this play out in other areas as well. My friend Annie decided to go after her health goals and reached out to me for support. I shared with her how nutritional cleansing has helped me and she got started. We live four hours apart, so my support comes through phone, text, social media, Zoom, and even snail mail.

On her first cleanse day, two of her local friends, Samantha and Renee, jumped on board and cleansed with her. These three amigos sailed through their day and came out on the other side feeling energized. In Annie's own words, "I feel very empowered and clear-headed... Wow, that's a first."

It was so neat to watch the thread of group texts of the three encouraging and supporting each other. Now, check out this beautiful second part:

Four hours away, two of my coaches and besties, Jim and Lucy joined me to send Annie, Samantha, and Renee additional prayers, positive energy, and support. We cheered them on through the day, evening, and into the following morning. It was a powerful collaboration that helped everyone take positive steps toward their health and overall feeling of success and teamwork.

Swolemates

My husband Jim and I share a passion as athletes. One passion is the bike. Others include strength training, kayaking, writing, and supporting our team to live life more abundantly.

Jim has trained me in the gym since 2007, sometimes one-on-one, some days in a group. In 2012, we met Sandra in a TRX class Jim was teaching. From day one, she was consistent. She showed up. Over the years, we became friends, beach buddies, and training buddies or "swolemates."

Swolemates play an essential part in your growth, improvement, and motivation. Together, the three of us became stronger, healthier athletes than any one of us could alone. It was often a conversation that didn't require words. It was an energy we felt and gave freely to each other.

On my weakest days, where all I could manage was to show up, Jim and Sandra were there, feeding me their energy, lifting me up, supporting and encouraging me. And knowing how much they were giving and putting in, how hard they were working, inspired me to dig a little deeper and work a little harder.

How about you? Who are two of your closest peeps? Have you asked them to join you on your journey? Have you linked arms with them? Have you invited them on your road to success?

Me to We

The way to spread the word and be a true ambassador of a healthy lifestyle is by living your life the best you can as a shining example. More importantly, you can encourage others your age and in your personal network to do the same. It is important to take care of yourself early in life so that as you age, you already have the tools to feel just as vibrant in your 60s as you did in your 20s or 30s.

Accountability is crucial. Keeping your commitments to yourself is essential. Communicating with your family and friends and engaging in social media groups can reinforce the importance of being surrounded by like-minded people and help you to stay accountable.

People in your life are watching. They will see your transformation and reach out, asking how they can experience something similar. Success loves company. At some point, your healthy lifestyle will be a bit more on autopilot and it will become more about who you can inspire to live a healthy life.

As a former weightlifting champion, most of Jim's athletic life involved individual sports. Coaching others as a personal trainer and network marketing professional in the health and wellness industry helped him shift my focus away from himself and onto others. It removed the "I" out of his vocabulary and replaced it with "we." Just like he's passing on his lessons learned, he learned this from others. Specifically, his friend Haley. She is a "we" person, and Jim learns from her every time she opens her mouth. She teaches him "we" on a daily basis. When they're together, he listens to her words. He looks at her posts on social media. He reads what she writes to her audience. He follows her example and feels himself changing when he talks to people.

Active Relationships

Do you find yourself struggling to choose between exercise and all the other responsibilities in your life? As you look at your calendar, do you silently wish for one more hour every day?

If you are like most people, you live a very full if not overflowing life. You fill your day from beginning to end and yet still feel like you're falling short, letting important relationships and healthy living fall through the cracks. When it comes to managing your time, not only is it difficult to try to fit everything in, it is also exhausting and overwhelming.

Life can be a complicated juggling act as you attempt to schedule work obligations, family priorities, commitments to friends, and social functions into your weekly or monthly calendar. And rest, relaxation, and recreation? Who has time for that?

What if you didn't have to choose between exercise and spending time with friends? What if you learned to incorporate fitness into your most important relationships?

By weaving relationships into an active lifestyle, you can nurture two priorities into one time slot and make room for what matters. You get to spend time with people you love and live a more active and healthier lifestyle.

Healthy relationships can help you manage stress and even lower your susceptibility to depression. Yet traditionally, exercise and relationships are treated as two different priorities and are kept separate. You block out one time slot to exercise and another for the important people in your life. In addition, relationships are commonly built around food and alcohol in a sedentary manner.

It's time to change your perspective and simplify your life and your calendar. By combining the important relationships in your life with physical activity and movement, your overall health and wellness will improve and your stress levels will drop. You'll help yourself and your loved ones. As you partner and collaborate with others, you'll be improving your time management skills, building a more active lifestyle, and simplifying a busy life.

As you look at the relationships you want to maintain or improve, ask yourself a few questions. What do you love to do? What did you enjoy doing as a child? What does your partner, parent, sibling, child, or other family member love to do? What can you do together?

Here are six relationships you can weave into an active and healthy lifestyle:

- **Romantic Relationships**
  Perhaps your partner loves to golf and you are a cyclist. Agree to try each other's sport. You can teach each other or sign up to take a lesson. Dates can be a sunrise or sunset walk, a day on the golf course, or a night out dancing.

- **Family Relationships**
  Family activities can include water balloon fights, trips to the playground, mini-triathlons, a game of badminton, or an obstacle course. Family exercise can even be centered around a home or yard project. Holiday or family get-togethers can include a game of frisbee, bocce ball, a walk after a meal, or a canoe or paddleboat ride at a local park.

- **Spiritual Relationships**
  Consider that your spiritual relationship doesn't have to be done sitting or even indoors. You can take your prayer and meditation time outdoors on a walk, or practice yoga. You can enjoy kayaking or rowing across a serene lake as the sun rises, or snowshoe through a winter field as the sun sets, enjoying the miracle of nature all around you.

- **Friendships**
  Grab a friend and visit the batting cages one night, and try yoga another. You can hike a mountain, go for a run, meet at the gym or go bowling. Head to the lake and rent a kayak or stand-up paddleboard. With enough friends, you can even form a soccer or softball team.
- **Work Colleagues**
  To nurture work relationships, consider a local charity event that involves walking, biking, or golf. For those more adventurous, you could experience a team-building event such as a low or high ropes course.
- **Relationship with Yourself**
  Finally, don't neglect the important relationship you have with yourself. Time alone to reflect and refresh can be done walking, running, hiking, horseback riding, biking, gardening, snowshoeing, or skiing.

Walking, hiking, miniature golf, climbing walls, trampoline parks, skating, snowshoeing, skiing, dancing, beach volleyball, frisbee, and bike riding are a few more ideas to explore together with your partner, family, friends, even co-workers.

Creating more time in your busy life with active relationships is a three-step process:

1. **Prioritize your relationships.**
   For some of you, your spiritual relationship will be the top priority. For others, you may be in a season of building your career, so nurturing your work relationships will rank highest. If your children are young, family time may be of most critical need. If you have aging parents, spending time with them may be of utmost importance.

2. **Set a Timeframe**
   The second step is to set a goal for the amount of time you want to allot to each relationship. Time to yourself or your family may require a daily time slot, whereas time with friends and co-workers may be a weekly, bi-weekly, or even monthly occurrence.

3. **Schedule It**
   On Sunday evening, look at your week and month ahead. For each relationship, begin to plan your schedule, adding in a date night, family event, time with friends, and work obligations. Don't forget to build in time for yourself or to nurture your spiritual relationship. Put it in writing. If your calendar is on your computer or phone, be sure to print it out and put it in a place where the entire family can see it. Set reminders on your phone so you don't forget, and review

your calendar daily. While it's ok to be flexible, it's not acceptable to cancel on the important people in your life, yourself included.

As you get creative with combining your relationships with an active lifestyle, you'll find you have fewer obligations and more time for what's important. As you simplify your life with some of these small changes, you'll be surprised at the extra time you find in your schedule for both exercise and the people you love.

Willpower Only Goes So Far

Choosing a healthy lifestyle is a daunting task. According to the Centers for Disease Control and Prevention, 42%–73% of Americans are obese or overweight. Unfortunately, around 80% of people who lose weight will gain it back within one year.[6]

On most days, you have the willpower and discipline to say "no." The trouble is, we have a limited number of "no's" to hand out each day. We say no once. Twice. Three times. Eventually, even the strongest person will run out of no's. When it is to the same person over the same food group at the same party three times in a row, well that's just plain aggravating. And, let's call it what it is: food bullying.

Losing weight and living a healthy lifestyle is a hero's journey. It is not for the faint of heart and there is no room for the people pleaser. A hero is a person who goes out and achieves great deeds on behalf of a group, tribe, civilization, or even on behalf of themselves or their family. Being as healthy as you possibly can be is a benefit to everyone in your life and makes you a hero to yourself and everyone around you.

People in your life may not be on the same journey as you when it comes to health and eating. They may live by an alternative philosophy of "eat dessert first; life is uncertain." And in living by such a philosophy, they want company. They want you to join them and they will ask again, and again, and again. They may say things like:

- "Oh, come on. One bite won't hurt you."
- "You're no fun anymore since you don't eat sweets / drink wine."
- "But I made this especially for you."

You can choose today to be true to yourself. Stay aware and focused on your goals and dreams so that when you say "yes" to please others, you are not disappointing yourself in the process.

Here are a few tips for saying no, being your own hero, and avoiding the people pleaser behaviors that derail you from your healthy lifestyle:

- **Say no**: Say no politely but firmly. "No, thank you. I'm taking steps to improve my health and that is not part of my plan."

- **Be firm:** Sometimes you need a firmer stance with yourself and others: "No, thank you. I don't eat that."
- **Set boundaries:** Let people know you love spending time with them but you are making changes for the benefit of your health and you won't be eating sugar / alcohol / gluten / ice cream / French fries anymore.
- **People don't know. Educate them:** People will admire your finished results but they may not have any idea of the time and hard work that is required with exercise as well as the discipline to cook and eat healthily. They don't know the process. We can make things easier by educating them and bringing it to their awareness.
- **Use your voice:** Recognize that what you eat or don't eat is YOUR choice. You have a voice and you can use it. What someone does with your yes or no is up to them. It's not on you. Release the guilt.
- **Call people on their crap:** You can do this with love. You can turn the tables on your loved ones by asking why it's so important to them that you eat what they are eating or have made. Say it with a smile on your face and then close your mouth. Wait for their reply. This can be a great stall technique and it gives you time to remember the steps above.
- **Nurture relationships another way:** If a relationship has always been about a meal or wine or dessert, let the other person know that you will be taking a break temporarily until you hit your goals. Ask if there is another way you can support the relationship without food. Perhaps a walk, exercise, hobby, or learning something new together.
- **People feel threatened:** Realize that sometimes the people closest to you feel threatened over the possibility of you changing. They will actively sabotage you to keep you from changing because they fear you will judge them or not like them anymore. Make your goals known to them and explain how much you would appreciate their help and how much you would value them.

YOUR TURN

Who in my life will offer me support, encouragement, and accountability toward my health and fitness goals?

_____

Who in my life will most likely sabotage my efforts toward my health and fitness goals?

_____

CHAPTER 4

Habits and Rules

AFTER MY HYSTERECTOMY, I took the recommended six weeks off and then returned to life as I knew it before surgery. Physically, I was fine, but I was exhausted. It felt like my emotions and my energy were on a roller-coaster ride. I had jumped back into my life at full speed and intensity. It was too much too soon. In the past, pushing harder was all I knew. Now, I couldn't.

In the weeks and months that followed, I sank deeper and deeper into my pity party and depression. My body, mind, and spirit had been through a trauma. I had to allow myself time to grieve and heal. But there came a point when I decided it was time to reclaim my joy and step back into my life boldly. I went to work on my mindset and habits.

Just like wellness is the result of deliberate effort and thought is a spiritual activity that must be consciously, systematically, and constructively directed, you must be intentional with your thoughts and your habits. What you consistently do on a daily basis determines or shapes your life. Bad habits (habits that do not serve you) and good habits (habits that serve you) are both built the exact same way: they are simply what you do consistently over time.

Learn to observe yourself. What do you do, without question or without much thought, on a routine basis? Observe everything, from the moment you wake up to the moment you go to sleep, and even observe your sleep patterns. What are the things you do automatically without even thinking?

These are the habits that you have built. Which ones support who you are and which ones support where you want to be (your goals and dreams)? When you observe yourself, it becomes easy to see what actions (habits) support your goals, and what actions (habits) lead you away from them. It becomes obvious what actions maintain your bliss and what actions steal your bliss.

Have a Plan

A healthy lifestyle involves change, and any plans for change are made with the left brain or the logical side of your brain. Plans are executed by the right side of your brain or your emotional side. Logic builds a plan, but your feelings execute it.

Safeguards must be put in place in the form of rules, which are consistently reinforced with healthy lifestyle decisions. The concept of not deviating from your long-term goals to get short-term satisfaction seems pretty straightforward. It's simple, but not always easy unless you practice.

First, let's recognize that you develop your meal plan with the part of your brain that is the most logic-based. But during the implementation of your plan, the part of our brain that is most influential is the feeling or emotional part. And your feelings can sabotage the best of intentions.

I am the first to admit that the best-laid plans can falter with emotions and feelings. But having no plan at all leaves your decisions based mostly on your emotions and feelings. This can be disastrous.

You must make decisions with the logical part of your brain and have a definite daily plan to execute. Do not begin your day not knowing exactly what you are going to eat throughout the day or your feelings will override your plan when life gets in the way or your day takes you on an unexpected course.

The new or future you—the healthier version of you— lives in your old world with constant reminders of old decisions and behaviors, and the same people you were comfortable having them with. During your journey to reach your goals, you constantly are faced with temptations to draw you back into poor eating decisions. If your goal is to eat healthier, lose weight, have more energy, perform better, or simply think more clearly, then you have to change your old decisions, habits, and behaviors that you are often much more comfortable with and replace them with new decisions, habits, and behaviors that are in alignment with your new goals. In the beginning, when you are first implementing changes, it is more difficult, but with time, practice and consistency, it will get easier.

Let's look at some of these temptations and pitfalls:

You make a promise to yourself to transform your life by sticking to your plan and you find yourself constantly facing dilemmas and compromising. Some of the reasons you get drawn back into making less than optimal choices include the following:

- Comfort foods are quick and easy to obtain when you're hungry or craving.
- Comfort foods offer a distraction from pain or discomfort.
- Your old "go-to" foods are familiar.

- Vending machines are everywhere.
- Rest stops often do not offer much in terms of healthy food.
- Fast-food restaurants are on every corner on your way home from work, and they call your name when you are exhausted and don't feel like cooking after a hard day.
- Favorite restaurants offer a reward for a good week or a balm after a hard week.
- Airline foods appear at the exact moment the monotony of the flight is starting to get to you.
- Snack foods left out at work surround you. Your co-workers don't want to leave temptation at home so they bring it into the office.
- Recreational and social eating where we nurture relationships around a meal.
- Parties filled with tempting drinks, desserts, and finger food (just one bite won't hurt, right?).
- Friends inviting you over and wanting to feed you, even after you've said no, multiple times.
- You feeling the need to feed friends, even if it's out of alignment with your goals.
- Celebratory eating for birthdays, weddings, and holidays.
- Business meals where you have no control over the menu.
- Using food or alcohol as medication—to soothe or calm yourself.
- Eating to distract yourself from pain or discomfort.
- Eating to feel full or avoid feeling empty.
- Numbing yourself to slow down your brain and feel more at ease.
- Physiological cravings because you are at a nutritional deficit.

Finally, you are often confronted by the food industry, which seduces you to buy cheaply produced processed foods that are made in a manner to increase profits and presented in a manner to get you to make a poor decision and crave them over and over again. These processed foods contain

- built-in food addictions such as salt, sugar, MSG, artificial sweetener, and fats, which cause your brain to produce dopamine, giving you comfort and making you want to eat these foods more and more often;
- wheat, which contains a protein called gliadin that makes us hungrier and increases cravings.

Only with a pre-thought-out plan can we make the best logical decisions each day, without being compromised by emotions and feelings. You must learn to negotiate all pitfalls in advance by having a plan.

Plan each day in advance, ideally the night before. Remove as many decisions as you can to cleanly execute your plan. Plan out your breakfast, lunch, dinner, as well as two healthy snacks to have mid-morning and mid-afternoon. Schedule twenty minutes of your lunch hour to go for a walk or climb the stairs in your building.

Decide Ahead of Time

Sometimes maintaining your healthy lifestyle requires you to decide ahead of time how you will respond in certain situations. You can set rules or declarations that are decisions made ahead of time for your own good, or toward the achievement of a goal. A few examples are

- I always take the stairs.
- I always park a large distance from the door at the mall. Even in the rain.
- I only check my personal email once per day.
- I limit my time on social media to 30 minutes.
- I work out six days per week.
- I schedule my workouts before 4 p.m.
- I work out with a buddy at least once per week.
- I will skip the alcohol, appetizer, and dessert while eating out.
- I will not add salt to my food.
- I will prepare my lunch at least four days per week.
- I will not hit the snooze button.
- I will turn off all electronics at least an hour before bed.
- I will go to bed 15 minutes earlier this week.

Can you imagine the difference it could make in your life to simply decide some of these things ahead of time instead of depending on how you are feeling in the moment when you are faced with a choice?

Think about when you get together with friends. You are so close to your goal weight, and you know that wine or dessert will derail you. Decide ahead of time.

Headed out to lunch or dinner? Look at the menu and decide on a healthy choice ahead of time what you will order. It is *so* much easier than in the moment when you get caught up in the excitement of seeing family or friends, or what others are having.

The beauty of setting rules and deciding ahead of time is that in a short period of time, they become a familiar, comfortable part of your healthy lifestyle.

What Is Best for Me

When it comes to life's decisions, life is not about finding yourself. It's more about creating yourself.

Every day you are presented with choices; decisions about what you are doing and how it impacts your body and your health. Everything that you ingest, regardless of the reason, everything that comes in contact with our skin (intentional or unintentional), everything you breathe into your body will affect you by either leaving you the same, better, or worse.

Why is this important? Because you are a perishable item and should live accordingly. Sometimes, you are making tough choices, such as, "If I do this to help this concern, what is the impact on this other concern, or will a different concern develop?" In other words, if I eat this because of these reasons, what is the impact on these other aspects of my life? If I take this drug for this reason, what are the side effects and what price will I pay?

To find the best answer to these tough questions, ask yourself: What is best for me? How you answer this question has a lot to do with your goals.

If you have a goal such as optimizing your health, reaching your ideal power-to-weight ratio, performing at your best, optimizing your intensity-to-recovery ratio, ensuring you age gracefully and without metabolic morbidity (the absence of health and wellbeing), or simply to inspire others that they can achieve and maintain a high state of wellness, then "What is best for me?" is one of the toughest questions that you can ask.

Ironically, sticking to your dreams, goals, and resulting decisions and actions holds you to the highest and most stringent standards. It has a lot to do with the premise of "do as I do" and having the resolve to set an example and hold yourself to a standard to maintain the integrity of your message.

With that in mind, make sure you understand that answers are not always found in other questions like:

- What will be easiest?
- What will be convenient?
- What would be the most enjoyable?
- What would be the most socially convenient?
- What would be easiest for others to understand and accept?
- What would be the most socially inclusive?
- What is in front of me right now?
- What is everyone else doing?
- What would give me the greatest short-term satisfaction?
- What is fastest?
- What is available?
- What is in my comfort zone?

- What can I do that requires no thought?
- What would make me feel good right now?
- What would make my mind stop spinning?
- What would help me go to sleep?
- What would stop me from feeling uncomfortable?
- What would make me feel full?
- What am I craving?

What is tough about the question of "What is best for me?" is that it requires an absolute answer. Not what's best in this situation, what's best right now, or what's better or, my favorite cop-out, "everything is cool in moderation." The problem with moderation is that you are getting mountains of hazardous stuff in moderation in your everyday foods, skincare, household cleaners, and personal hygiene products that you come in contact with and breathe in, intentional or unintentional, much of which is labeled deceptively.

The answer to the question "What is best for me?" starts with your dream of a better, healthier you. When these dreams are written down, they become goals. How big should your health goal be? This often requires re-examining and re-learning past beliefs that have not gotten you where you want to be or enabled a transformation you want.

Is This Decision Helping or Hurting the Future Me?

Your beliefs influence your thoughts and your thoughts influence your feelings. Thus your beliefs, thoughts, and feelings influence your actions. Your actions create consequences and in turn, you develop and build new beliefs.

So you have beliefs that influence thoughts; thoughts that influence feelings; feelings that influence actions; actions that have consequences; and consequences that build or reinforce your beliefs. This can spiral around and build or reinforce negatively or positively. It can move you either towards or away from your goals.

Your thoughts, beliefs, feelings, actions, and results define your comfort zone, which is where your habits reside. You build your comfort zone, either consciously or on autopilot.

Take for example the unhealthy cycle when it comes to diet and nutrition: when you eat like crap, you feel like crap and when you feel like crap, you eat like crap. You can't wait until you feel good to eat well, you must take action and start eating better in order to feel better. This begins with a change in your decisions or your actions. By changing your actions, not only do you get different results, you think different thoughts, which influences your beliefs and feelings. So the cause is you take action to eat healthier and the effect is that you get better results, think more positively, and feel better.

You must identify the actions that are helping you and reinforce them, and you must identify the actions that are hurting you and replace them with better ones. If you want to change your life it begins by changing your mind on purpose and with intention.

First, decide what is important to you and why (revisit chapter one if needed). Then, make changing your unhealthy habits a top priority. When changing unhealthy habits is an 8, 9, or 10 on a scale of 1 to 10 in regard to importance, then you will begin to build your new comfort zone. When you spend the three to six weeks necessary being uncomfortable, you give yourself a chance to build a new comfort zone— a comfort zone that serves you and your goals for living a healthy lifestyle.

A simple way to discover where you need change is to ask yourself, "Is what I am doing—my actions—moving me toward my goals to a better place, or away from my goals to a worse place? Is this decision helping or hurting the future me?"

Your Aunt Zelda just offered you her famous peach cobbler. Before answering, ask yourself, "Will eating this move me toward my goals or away from them?"

Your co-workers decide to go out for happy hour, for the third night in a row. Ask yourself, "Will having an alcoholic beverage move me toward my goals, or away from them? Can I go out and socialize and abstain from drinking alcohol, at least until I reach my goals?"

The alarm goes off at 0-dark-thirty and you consider hitting the snooze button and skipping your morning workout. "Will skipping my workout move me to a better or worse place?"

These small actions done with consistency over time can be the key to your successful transformation.

I Don't Eat That

Along your journey of building a consistent healthy lifestyle, you will be faced with temptations that threaten to throw you off your plan.

"I don't eat that" is a simple statement that draws a line in the sand. It is designed to take a personal stand, particularly in what could be compromising social situations that serve or display food in conflict with your nutritional goals. This statement publicly strengthens your resolve to stick to your healthy lifestyle and meal plan while allowing other people to hold you accountable.

At our first meal at a resort in Costa Rica, I told the waiter I was gluten-free. I was essentially saying, "I don't eat that (gluten)." The word quickly spread to other servers and even other restaurants, and for the entire week, the staff helped and supported my gluten-free meal plan.

This statement comes in handy in social settings. At a restaurant, tell your waiter not to bring you the bread or chips because "I don't eat that (empty carbs)." At a party, decline the cheese platter because "I don't eat that (dairy)." At an event, ask for your portion to be prepared plainly because "I don't eat that (heavy sauces ladened with fat)."

"I don't eat ___" is a great rule and statement where you can fill in the blank with a multitude of things—anything that you know will sabotage your healthy lifestyle or take you off track and further from your goals, rather than closer.

- I don't eat cupcakes.
- I don't eat unplanned meals or snacks.
- I don't eat bread during my evening meal.
- I don't drink coffee.
- I don't drink my calories.
- I don't eat after 7:00 p.m.

Some of the foods that derail you and that you may want to eliminate—even temporarily—from your healthy lifestyle include alcohol, sugar, salt, bread, cookies, cakes, muffins, pizza, burgers, and fried foods. Simply adopt the language and mindset of "I don't eat that." If you feel the need to further clarify, you can say, "That doesn't align with my current goals for a healthy lifestyle."

Recognize that your palate or what you desire and crave is a habit and a choice. You develop and choose to keep them or let them die. These are decisions you make and reinforce.

Use this statement as a daily affirmation and a tool to build better habits. When confronted with food items that do not serve your goals, state out loud, "I don't eat that." When you think about food items that do not serve you, state out loud, "I don't eat that." Don't worry if there are people around you. There is no need to be embarrassed. In fact, if they look at you funny or ask you what you mean, share with them your health goals and how you are creating healthier habits and a stronger mindset. Just speaking it out loud and sharing it with someone, even if that person is a stranger, will reinforce your plan and decision to living a lifestyle, similar to when you share your "why."

If you are offered food items that do not serve you and you feel hesitant, right away, before you falter, state out loud, "I don't eat that." This is a mental muscle, and the more you flex it the more powerful it will get. You will strengthen the habit of staying the course and building your resolve.

Give yourself time to allow healthy foods to replace those not-so-healthy foods. Practice saying no to these foods that aren't helping you live as healthy as you possibly can. Focus on the great-tasting foods that move you toward your goals.

Allow your beliefs, thoughts, feelings, behaviors, and results toward foods to change and over time, you will build new healthy habits. Let the desires and cravings for these food items that take you away from your goals die within you and replace them with those that move you toward your goals.

Food Is Fuel

To an athlete, food is fuel. There is never a time when you are not preparing for, competing in, or recovering from your sport. Athletes are disciplined to eat in a way that is consistent with their goals.

Just like when you have a weight loss goal, if you have a fitness goal then it is best to have a plan and strategy in place to fuel your body. You need to ingest the required nutrients daily to stay healthy, have the energy to perform and recover optimally, and support all vital bodily functions necessary to sustain your athletic efforts.

A self-awareness tool is to pause before eating and ask yourself, "Why am I eating this?"

The best answer is, "It's on my eating plan, it meets my standards as a clean fuel, and it will get me closer to my goals."

Some less than stellar answers include:

- I am medicating with food.
- It will make me feel better.
- I'm anxious and overwhelmed. I want to feel numb.
- If I eat this, I will calm down by feeling full or satisfied.
- I want to eat this so I do not feel so emotionally empty.
- I need or deserve this.
- I'm having emotional or psychological cravings.
- It is comfort food.
- It is a trigger food.
- It is my routine. I eat ice cream or a cookie or drink a glass of wine before bed or with a meal.
- I am bored. I eat when I have nothing to do or I'm under-stimulated.
- I am using food to lower my brainwaves. I need to quiet my mind and get out of this over-excited state.
- I am too _____ (angry, lonely, hungry, bored, depressed, tense, anxious, unhappy, tired, overworked, stressed, busy, frustrated, intense, apathetic, exhausted, etc.).
- I am eating recreationally for entertainment, socially, or holiday binging.

Before you eat, remember that the best answer as to why you are eating is, "It's on my eating plan, it meets my standards as a clean fuel, and it will get me closer to my goals." Any other answer will have a direct impact on accomplishing your goal.

How You Do One Thing

How you do one thing is how you do everything. When you can sit in the discomfort of losing weight or transforming your body, you can sit in the discomfort elsewhere. If you can transform your body, you can transform your life.

In the first few days, weeks, or months where you embrace change, you may feel uncomfortable. But at some point after weeks of consistency, your mind turns. You're still uncomfortable, but it gets easier to just get through it. With more consistency come better results and more momentum.

Most of your discomfort lies in the fact that your new behavior is not familiar. You're used to and more comfortable with your old behaviors.

I have run a marathon, climbed a 14er, and ridden a century. Each time, I faced the desire to quit. The battle was between my mind and body.

Every spring, after taking a few months off, I begin to build my mileage up. I start with a ten-mile ride, and the last two miles suck. The next time I add five miles, and the last four miles suck. But my body and mind remember those first ten. It's like they are telling each other "Hey. Yeah. We can do this. We've done this before."

Think back to a time in your life when you experienced success. It could be an achievement like you graduated from high school, ran a 5k, quit drinking, received a promotion, or made your bed this morning. Think about how proud you were. Focus on your strengths and the positive, and you'll face your transformation with a better, more optimistic perspective.

Four Things Successful People Do

For several years when Jim was a finalist and runner-up and then when I became a finalist, I was surrounded by people that had successfully accomplished a goal of transforming their body, health, and / or their life. I observed them closely, knowing that they beat the odds and achieved success where others failed. I learned that success requires four things:

- the courage to start;
- the discipline to keep going;

- practice;
- daily consistent action to get it done.

In 2017 Jim and I attended our company's annual celebration in Las Vegas, where Jim was awarded runner-up in that year's challenge. This sixteen-week transformation challenge requires you to submit before and after photos and a short essay. There are three challenges per year, and each one results in five finalists. Jim was one of fifteen finalists out of 35,000 participants for the year. Jim not only redefined healthy aging (at age 65) and transformed his body, he won $13,000 and two all-expenses-paid trips to Las Vegas and Costa Rica (for me too). Pretty outstanding results. I call that success. Two years later I became a finalist, winning $3,000 and an all-expenses-paid trip for two to Costa Rica.

One of the most remarkable aspects to me is that for the entire year in 2017, over 109,000 people started the challenge.

35,000 finished.

Only 32% of the people that started this sixteen-week challenge actually finished it.

In studying the habits and mindset of the finalists over the years, I learned what these successful finishers have in common: courage, discipline, daily consistent action, and the commitment to finish.

1. **Courage**

   Whether you are starting a diet, exercise program, writing your first book, pursuing a dream or passion, improving your finances, or even starting a new relationship, courage is the step that moves you to action. Let's face it, we all struggle with procrastination from time to time. It's easy to say I'll start tomorrow, or Monday, or when I'm less busy or stressed. Sometimes we even put things off because we simply don't feel like doing them. The reality is, if we wait until we feel like it, we may never get anything done.

   I love the 5 Second Rule by Mel Robbins.[7] Basically, as soon as an idea comes to mind, you count backward from 5 and when you get to 1, you launch yourself into action: 5, 4, 3, 2, 1, GO. It is a tool that takes practice and can begin with something as simple as getting up in the morning. As soon as the alarm goes off (or you wake up), count backward from 5 and then launch yourself out of bed. This is a great way to reenergize your mornings.

2. **Discipline**

   Maybe starting isn't the hard part for you. You can start, and start, and start again, however, it's the continuation and sticking with something that you can sometimes struggle with. This is where discipline comes in. It cannot come from something external. It absolutely has to come from within. You have to know WHY you are doing something. Why is it important to you to be healthy? Why do you want to write a book? What will it feel like to grow your savings or investment account? When you keep your reason why at the forefront, you will find yourself making better decisions, creating more consistent daily habits, and practicing the discipline to keep going.

3. **Practice**
    Athletes know how much hard work and practice goes into improving in your sport. One thing all successful cyclists have in common is practice. They ride their bikes two, three, four times or more each week. They ride with groups, they practice hill climbing and sprinting. They know and follow the Law of Practice and the 5Ps: Perfect Practice Prevents Poor Performance.

    Years ago I participated and competed in a mini Triathlon camp. I remember telling my friend and coach Andrew, an elite triathlete, that the swim was my weakest link. He asked me, "How often do you practice?" My reply: "I don't." To which he said, "Exactly." I had been a runner for 24-plus years and then transitioned to the bike, which I fell in love with. I rode often and practiced my biking skills. The swim? Not so much. With practice comes improvement and ultimately, success.

4. **Daily Consistent Action**
    Success loves consistency. It does not always come from giant leaps, but from the daily consistent action toward a goal. Consistency builds momentum and keeps you moving forward. If your goal is weight loss, it will happen with what you do consistently, not once in a while. If it is to build financial wealth, it comes from consistent savings and investment. Have a book to finish or project at work? It will get done with consistent action.

    Once you know your reason for wanting to accomplish something, set a timeframe with deadlines and dates. This is where keep the finish in mind right from the start. If it is writing a book, the finish may be when you get the first draft to your editor, when you have the first printed copy in your hands, or when you have sold your first 100 copies. If your goal is about health or fitness, it may be when you release a certain amount of pounds, fit into a certain size, or run your first 5k.

Put the date in writing. Make it a challenge, but reasonable. Then work backward, chunking your goal into smaller bite-size pieces. Set small tasks that you can get done and feel good about, and work with daily consistent action.

I Persist Until I Succeed

I will persist until I succeed.
I was not delivered into this world into defeat, nor does failure course in my veins.
I am not a sheep waiting to be prodded by my shepherd.
I am a lion and I refuse to talk, to walk, to sleep with the sheep.
The slaughterhouse of failure is not my destiny.
I will persist until I succeed. [8]
~ Og Mandino, The Greatest Salesman in the World

In addition to having the courage to start, the discipline to keep going, practice, and daily consistent action, you will also require resilience. Failure and quitting cannot be part of your vocabulary or mindset.

Consider this: once you start backing down, it gets easier and easier to give up. When you quit the first time, it's hard. When you quit a second time, it gets easier. By the time you quit a third time, you don't even think about it. Quitting becomes a way of life.

What's the difference between thousands of people who quit versus the few who stick it out?

A decision.

Make the decision to never, never, never give up on your goals and dreams. Make a total commitment to never give up. Decide and commit to finish what you start.

Choose to persist until you succeed.

Cooking for Multiple Meals—Healthy Living Made Simple

I love being home and planning, prepping, and cooking fresh meals. However, let's face it, a great life can get full, and some days, we simply run out of time. And I've learned that if I go too long without a meal or snack, I become hangry.

HANGRY: When you are so hungry that your lack of food causes you to become angry, frustrated, or both.

Over the years, I've found a couple of tricks that help keep me on task with my healthy lifestyle so that I don't sabotage my success. This way, a good, healthy, nutritious meal is only minutes away when I am hungry or past my mealtime or heading towards HANGRY.

- **Keep your freezer full**
  Stock your freezer with soups, veggie burgers, and frozen veggies. On my days at home, I love making soups, stews, veggie burgers, stud muffins, and protein balls. I always make at least a double batch and then I freeze them in individual servings to pull out for a quick meal or snack. Most of my soups are plant-based and always gluten-free, making them quite versatile. You can always add lean chicken. The soups pair great with a salad. You can also add potato, rice or noodles to make it heartier and boost up the calories.

- **Always make extra**
  Veggies, soup, salad, chicken, rice, quinoa—whatever you are cooking, make extra. You can either freeze, as in the case of soups and veggie burgers, or use later on in the week for lunch or repurpose for dinner.
  Are you grilling out tonight? Add some extra chicken to the grill to top off your salad for lunch tomorrow. You could also chop it up for chicken salad wrapped in your favorite lettuce leaf.
  Grilling or steaming veggies? Make extra. They will go great on top of a bed of greens or over rice or quinoa.
  Is quinoa or rice on the menu? Make extra. You can always pull out a soup to top it with, or a can of beans and salsa, or even tuna and Vegenaise®. They also make a great base for a breakfast bowl topped with your favorite berries, seeds, and milk or non-dairy milk substitute.

- **Pack away your leftovers first**
  This one comes from a conversation I had with my friend Nathalie. She said even when she makes extra food, her family (she has growing boys of the teenage variety) scarfs it up at dinner. To solve this dilemma, before you sit down to dinner, pack a serving or two away for your lunch this week.
  Making a dinner salad? While you are building it in a family-size bowl, have two side containers right next to it and build two smaller salads along with the larger one. One for dinner tonight, and two for lunch this week.

- **Fresh is great, but in a pinch, frozen veggies will do**
  I love fresh veggies that I grow myself or pick up at a local farmers market. But some days you run out of time, and the

garden isn't ready, and you miss the health food store, and its two days before the CSA delivers. This is where frozen veggies come in handy for a quick soup, side dish, or stir-fry.

Plus, frozen spinach, broccoli, onions, and peppers all work great in an egg scramble. Great for breakfast, a mid-morning snack, or paired with potatoes for a breakfast-for-dinner meal.

- **Dried beans are great but keep a few canned (BPA free) on hand**

  I love dried beans, but you really have to plan ahead to soak and cook them for most recipes. That's why it's helpful to have a pantry with a few different varieties of beans. Chickpeas work great on a salad or roasted for a snack. Lima or black work well with quinoa or rice and salsa.

- **Meal replacement shakes**

  Perhaps my best tip is to have meal replacement shakes on hand. Meal replacement shakes are a healthy way of life. Quick and easy and oh so tasty. I eat five or six meals a day and, as much as I love to meal plan, prep, and cook, I also love my shakes.

  I always have one with me along with a shaker bottle, whether I'm just going out for a quick errand or on the road for a few hours. I usually have water with me as well, but if not, that is usually as close as the nearest gas station. It is a strange phenomenon that people have an aversion to a meal replacement shake but smoothies are commonly accepted, where you mix fruit, protein powder, and other options into a blender. But for me, I feel like I'm guessing at the right amounts to make sure I'm getting the right combination of protein, fats, and carbs. With my meal replacement shakes, I simply have to add water and I know, I'm getting a perfectly balanced meal or snack, designed by scientists and formulators that are much more knowledgeable, skilled, and experienced than me.

  Here are my standards for a great shake:
    - Substantial enough to be a meal replacement (approx. 240+ calories)
    - Protein should be a grade seven undenatured whey (from New Zealand preferably)
    - Plant-based shakes should be some combination of pea, hemp, mung bean, or brown rice protein
    - Low glycemic
    - High fiber
    - Free of gluten and soy
    - Contain vitamins and minerals
    - Contain probiotics and prebiotics
    - Contain active enzymes to aid digestion

- ○ No artificial flavoring, coloring, preservatives or chemicals
- ○ Taste great

Navigating Meals Out

If you find yourself eating out a lot, either for work or in your personal life, there are some things you can do to keep yourself on track and not derail your healthy lifestyle goals and plans.

Eat something healthy before and after the event so that you don't arrive at these situations hungry or you can remind yourself you have a healthy snack or meal waiting for you in the car. This is where that high protein, high fiber, nutritionally dense meal replacement shake comes in handy. This way, you're not starving when you sit down to socialize or network.

Stick to your workouts the day of and the day after your meal out. If possible, add in an extra walk.

Stay hydrated. Remember that thirst can be mistaken as hunger.

Decide ahead of time to skip alcohol, desserts, and / or appetizers. Enjoy a glass of water in a fancy glass with lime or olive.

Make a promise to yourself to not fill up on chips or bread.

Pace yourself. Eat slowly and chew thoroughly to give your body time to recognize when it's full. You may find you are bringing half your entree home.

If it's a mixer or buffet or casual party, show up late and bow out early and choose to pass on food altogether, while focusing on socializing or networking.

YOUR TURN

What goals do you have today?

_____

_____

What changes in direction does your life need?

_____

_____

Are your dreams coming closer or further away?

_____

What small step can you take today toward achievement?

_____

Transform

CHAPTER 5

Victim to Hero

SUCCESSFUL PEOPLE REALIZE THAT setbacks, disappointments, and problems are temporary. Tough times never last. Quitters view setbacks, disappointments, and problems as permanent. They lose hope, play the victim, lean into drama, blow things out of proportion, and talk about it until it becomes their story or mantra.

When you embrace a quitting mentality, you lose hope. You lose something you can rejoice about. You lose something that gives you strength. You lose something that renews your strength in times of need. Hope brings you peace and understanding, and attracts people who can't thrive without hope.

Successful people take responsibility. There is no blaming, complaining, or whining. They charge forward. They stop trying and they start doing. They choose perseverance in the face of adversity knowing that what the mind can conceive and believe, the body can achieve.

This mental toughness is a choice you make. It is something you build within yourself. It's not a gift that only a select number of people have or are born with. It involves using your mind to infuse positive thoughts and actions into your life that reinforce your efforts and goals. When you embark on a healthy lifestyle, sometimes you skip the most important step: preparing your mind. And your mind is just another aspect that you train with intention.

When you choose to approach a healthy lifestyle from a logical standpoint instead of an emotional reaction, when you decide to change your body as an act of self-love, and when you accept that failure is part of every success, you'll begin to understand that power is found in the choices you make and the actions you take.

When you take the time to define your goals and get in touch with why you want to live your healthiest life, when you can recognize your own triggers, obstacles, and ways that you self-sabotage, when you seek out support instead of solitude in your quest, and when you recreate your habits with intention, you'll move from a victim mindset to the hero in your own life story.

Moving from victim to hero will require that you keep your promises, tune out the naysayers and voice of self-doubt, let go of your past and your inner Charlie Brown, and take action. These are not tools of overnight success, but of a great adventure where you persist until you succeed.

Keep Your Promise

Peer pressure and social expectations lead you to say yes when you want to say no. You worry about disappointing others, yet what hurts more is when you disappoint yourself. Each and every time you do something that is out of alignment with the goal you set for the promise you made, you make it easier to do again and again. When you keep your word, you build the muscle and the mindset that you always keep your promises.

To make and keep your promise may be the most important decision you nurture. To not keep your promise is to reinforce the pattern of failure.

How often do you make a promise? A promise could be as simple as
- I'll take the trash out after dinner.
- I'll do the dishes.
- I'll call you to set up a lunch date.
- I'll have it done by Friday.
- I'll make it to my kid's game at the beginning, instead of the end.

Do you keep your promises? Or is there a never-ending list of excuses you rattle off for not doing what you said you'd do?

What about all the promises you make to yourself:
- I'll eat healthier this week.
- I'll cut back on my drinking.
- I'll quit smoking.
- I'll write my book.
- I'll start singing again.
- I'll go to the gym I joined.
- I'll clean out the junk drawer.
- I'll stay present with my kids.
- I won't bring work home.

Whether you are making a commitment to someone else or to yourself, it is critical that you do what you say you'll do. Otherwise, it's better to not say it at all in the first place.

"...when we start something and do not complete it, or make a resolution and do not keep it, we are forming the habit of failure; absolute, ignominious failure. If you do not intend to do a thing, do not start; if you do start, see it through even if the heavens fall; if you make up your mind to do something, do it; let nothing, no one, interfere..."9
~ Charles Haanel, Part Four: The Master Key System

You may be thinking, what's the big deal? So what if I didn't take the trash out when I said I would?

The big deal is that success and keeping your word are found in your daily actions. Remember, how you do one thing is how you do everything. Every time you say you're going to do something and you don't, you are forming the habit of failure. While your lack of keeping your word may affect many people, the most important person you're hurting or disappointing is you.

At the end of the day, you have to face yourself in the mirror and ponder whether you were true to yourself. If the answer is anything other than "hell yeah," then you are the one who's hurting you. The guilt and shame that comes with disappointing yourself carry into every nook and cranny of your life, eroding your self-confidence with every yes that was meant to be a no.

In the months prior to a significant birthday, Jim made a promise to himself: that he would be as healthy as he could possibly be by that birthday. He made it measurable by adding a weight loss goal. He followed through using a healthy diet and workout schedule with daily consistent action.

Every day he was faced with opportunities and decisions to go off track. Friends and family would encourage him to make an exception "just this one time." After all, one time won't hurt, right?

The reality is, one time will hurt.

Each and every time you do something that is out of alignment with the goal you set for the promise you made, you make it easier to do again and again. When you keep your word, you build the muscle and the mindset that you always keep your promises.

Jim didn't give in to temptation—and trust me when I say he had them. He kept the promise he made to himself. In the days before his birthday, he hit his goal: He looked and felt as healthy as he possibly could be.

As his wife, I'm extremely proud of him and grateful for his commitment to his health. I also know how proud he is of himself for keeping his word. He is a promise keeper and he inspires me to be one too.

Voice of Truth

During my first sixteen-week challenge, I shared my dream and goal with a group of women at a supper club gathering. One woman, who I considered a friend, said to me, "It's not like you can win. You don't have enough weight to lose. What kind of transformation can you possibly have?"

At the time, my goal and dream weren't to lose weight. My goal was to build a strong, muscular body so that my outsides matched how I felt on the inside. Even as I shared this with her, I could tell she still had her doubts. It was hard to accept the fact that someone I considered a close confidant and supporter was speaking to me with negativity and skepticism.

It's hard enough to battle your own voice of self-doubt, without adding in the voice of those who unknowingly—or knowingly—try to sabotage you. Building a strong mindset will require you to ignore the voices of the naysayers, the bullies, and all those who doubt your success or believe that the odds of winning are against you. You will have to tune out the voice that threatens to steal your belief so that you can tune in to the voice of truth.

> *Oh, what I would do to have*
> *the kind of faith it takes*
> *to climb out of this boat I'm in,*
> *onto the crashing waves.*
> *To step out of my comfort zone*
> *into the realm of the unknown where Jesus is*
> *and He's holding out His hand.*
> *But the waves are calling out my name*
> *and they laugh at me.*
> *Reminding me of all the times*
> *I've tried before and failed.*
> *The waves they keep on telling me*
> *time and time again, "Boy, you'll never win. You'll never win."*
> *But the voice of truth tells me a different story.*
> *The voice of truth says, "Do not be afraid"...*
> *Out of all the voices calling out to me*
> *I will choose to listen and believe the voice of truth.*
> *~ "Voice of Truth" recorded by Casting Crowns, written by Mark*
> *Hall and Steven Curtis Chapman (2003)*

Isn't that what the hero's journey is all about? You're like Peter in the boat on the Sea of Galilee (from Matthew 14:22–33). You want to stay in the boat, not because it's comfortable, but because it's familiar. And yet at the same time, your heart yearns for something more. Something great.

74

It longs to live a life of health and wellness, passion, and purpose. It longs to live life more abundantly.

"You are here to live as your highest expression. You are here to be your beautiful, empowered, sacred, holy self without apology, without explanations, without trepidation. Let us see her. And let us all be changed by the power of her divine confidence and courage."[10]
~ Debbie Ford

The boat represents our comfort zone. Jesus calling to us, to step out onto the water into the "realm of the unknown" is the Herald calling us. It's our dreams and our soul calling us.

Will we answer the call?

When you picked up this book you said yes to the call. Every chapter, every page, every paragraph, and every word that you've read since then, you've been accepting the call to live a healthy lifestyle, whatever you defined that to be for you personally back in chapter one.

However, every hero's journey hits a wall and an abyss before you experience transformation, atonement, and your beautiful, miraculous self with your new mindset and set of healthy habits. In the stages immediately before the abyss, you experience challenges, temptations, and doubt.

Suddenly, instead of thinking like a hero, you are doubting like a victim with thoughts like:

- Perhaps I got it wrong.
- Perhaps that healthy lifestyle isn't really meant for me.
- Perhaps I dreamed too big.
- Perhaps I can't lose weight after all.

The temptation to shrink your dreams becomes this thundering voice in your head.

"Our deepest fear is not that we are inadequate. Our deepest fear is that we are powerful beyond measure. It is our light, not our darkness that most frightens us. We ask ourselves, Who am I to be brilliant, gorgeous, talented, fabulous?"[11]
~ Marianne Williamson

During these times, the better questions to ask yourselves are

- What am I hanging on to so hard that I don't want, that prevents me from having what I do want?
- What am I pretending not to know?
- If I could not fail, what would I do?
- If money, time, and health were not an issue, what would I do tomorrow, and with who?

And perhaps the best question to ask ourselves comes from Marianne Williamson:

"Who am I to be brilliant, gorgeous, talented, fabulous? Actually, who are you not to be?

You are a child of God. Your playing small does not serve the world. There is nothing enlightened about shrinking so that other people won't feel insecure around you. We are all meant to shine, as children do. We were born to make manifest the glory of God that is within us. It's not just in some of us; it's in everyone.

And as we let our own light shine, we unconsciously give other people permission to do the same. As we are liberated from our own fear, our presence automatically liberates others."[12]

Og Mandino reinforces this idea in Scroll IV of *The Greatest Salesman in the World:*

"I am nature's greatest miracle. I am not on this earth by chance. I am here for a purpose and that purpose is to grow into a mountain, not to shrink to a grain of sand. Henceforth will I apply all my efforts to become the highest mountain of all and I will strain my potential until it cries for mercy."[13]

The following are a few questions to revisit at this point in your journey:

- What is my personal health goal?
- Why do I want to achieve that particular goal?
- What am I willing to give up to have the life of my dreams and to step toward the healthy version of my life?
- What do I want now versus what do I want most?

- What unhealthy habits do I need to let go of?
- If I give up fear and doubt, would I receive love and faith?

Overall, you have a choice to listen to the voice of powerlessness, hopelessness, helplessness, and insecurity, or tune into the voice of acceptance, power, confidence, courage, strength, forgiveness, and grace. You get to choose which voice guides you.

There will be times when you hear the voice of fear and doubt. Sometimes it gets loud and threatens to take you under like a riptide. With practice, you can learn to tune it out. A few tools that will help include meditation, the Law of Substitution, and a kudos file or flashcards.

- **Meditation**
  As you sit each day in quiet stillness, thoughts of doubt may come up. The practice of meditation is to let them go. Like a revolving door, just keep sending them on their way. As you sit and relax

first your physical body and eventually your mind, you will learn to replace the voice of fear and doubt with the voice of truth. You will come to understand that what you focus on grows, therefore it is essential that you forget those negative thoughts of self-doubt.

- **The Law of Substitution**

  It is impossible to think about two things at the same time. When a negative thought enters your mind, immediately think of something positive. Use any fond memory, previous accomplishment, or other pleasant thought.

- **Kudos File and Flashcards**

  Part of refocusing your mind toward the positive involves celebrating and remembering your own victories and strengths. When I was recovering from my hysterectomy and surgical menopause, two tools helped me restore a positive mindset: a kudos box and flashcards.

  Kudos is praise and honor received for an achievement. Saved greeting cards, notes, and awards can encourage you on your journey. You can keep them all in a kudos shoebox or in a folder on your computer, and when you're feeling sad, sift through them to lift your spirits.

  Flashcards created on index cards can increase your confidence. Start with writing out twenty achievements you are proud of, one per card. An achievement could be that you graduated from high school or you made your bed this morning. Add to your flashcards daily things you love about yourself and past victories. Examples can include you woke up this morning, learned to meditate, or started exercising. Flash through your cards daily. Do it when you first wake up, before you go to bed, after every meal, and whenever you start to feel sad. It doesn't matter how big or small the accomplishment is. The goal is to reinforce and celebrate victories. As you focus on your strengths and the positive, you'll feel your mood lightened and lifted.

Self-doubt may be the tiger you continue to wrestle with. As a finalist, Amazon best-selling author, wife, friend, daughter, and human being, I still battle times of fear, negativity, and self-doubt. It doesn't go away when you achieve some level of success. The tools above help me turn things around quickly so that I'm listening more to the voice of truth than to the naysayers or my inner critic.

Letting Go of Your Inner Charlie Brown

Charles Monroe Schulz (November 26, 1922—February 12, 2000), nicknamed Sparky, was an American cartoonist best known for the comic strip *Peanuts*, which featured the characters Charlie Brown and Snoopy, among others. He is widely regarded as one of the most influential cartoonists of all time.

As a child, during his formative years, Jim watched Snoopy, Charlie Brown and friends on TV, and read about their adventures in the Sunday comics.

For Charlie Brown, there was always something (often the same things you and I allow) standing in the way of the simple things that he wanted in life. The motivation was never the issue: he tried, and tried, and tried again. But each time he failed. He was never able to overcome his obstacles.

What were some of the simple things he wanted?

- To pitch a winning baseball game.
- To keep a kite in the air.
- To win a game of checkers.
- To successfully punt a football.

One particular comic stuck with Jim throughout his entire life, buried deep within his subconscious mind. It is an image of Charlie Brown, face down in between a rock and his sister Sally. The bubble caption above Charlie Brown reads, "Every day I trip over that rock!" The bubble caption above his younger sister Sally's head reads, "Why don't you move it?"

Throughout his life, Jim struggled over some of the same obstacles, each time asking himself, "Why don't you move it?" But every time he got the same answer: "I am a victim of circumstance." (Curly, *The Three Stooges*)

It took moving from feeling like a victim to taking responsibility and empowering himself to make changes to his habits and life; something Jim learned from another childhood television show: *The Wizard of Oz*. At the end of the movie, we learn that Dorothy had the power all along to get home, although throughout their journey she and her friends played the part of the victim, unaware of their own gifts and strengths.

Just like Dorothy, you, too, have the solutions within yourself to live a life of true health, love, laughter, and freedom. You are the hero you are looking for. You may dream of someone or something riding into your life to save you. But the best satisfaction is to rescue yourself. There is no need to give this power away. You are in charge. Don't give the responsibility away.

Take responsibility for your health by recognizing the decisions you make daily. Recognize where you can take control of your life. At this moment you can decide to not eat the cookie or reach for caffeine. You can decide to do whatever it takes to get to the gym or complete your workout. This falls in line with knowing the reason why you want to make a change toward better health, so that every decision you make is in line with that goal, dream, or purpose, and so you can make decisions that are life-affirming. In taking responsibility for your daily decisions, you will let go of your inner Charlie Brown.

Take Action

Was there ever a time in your life where you took action and it changed the course of your life? Action is the step that takes us closer to our goals, changes the direction of our lives, and makes dreams come true.

It's not the leap that gets you to the finish line of a marathon or even a 5k. It's the small action of signing up for the race. You don't sit down and write a manuscript in one day, it's the daily act of writing, even if only fifteen minutes or five pages at a time, that creates a book. It's not one large action that makes a dream come true, it's the millions of small actions and decisions along the way that get it started. Small changes done consistently will bring you success. In the pursuit of a healthy lifestyle, don't try to change everything at once. Make small, bite-size changes that you can maintain with consistency.

It's the decision made in a split-second that starts the forward motion. It tells your mind you are serious. It doesn't matter what you've done or haven't done or procrastinated in the past. One small action will begin to reprogram your brain and rebuild the blueprint that will move you forward toward the success you seek.

This is especially true with our health and fitness goals. You can have a goal to lose weight, run a 5k or get in the best shape of your life, but until you take action, it's only a wish.

Simple actions can get you started:
- Sign up for yoga or a spin class
- Register for a local 5k race
- Call a friend to set a date to ride, run or walk together
- Create a healthy grocery list
- Contact a personal trainer, nutritionist, or health coach

Any of these small steps put you in action. They start the momentum moving forward, closer to your goals.

Many years ago, I was in a relationship where my partner was angry, controlling, and did not treat me very well. Rant sessions were a daily occurrence, where he yelled, screamed, and complained about everything wrong in his life, and I was expected to just listen and commiserate. God forbid I look on the bright side or offer a solution. It was safer to simply stay quiet. One particular evening, I found myself tuning out, and five seconds of action changed the course of my life. He looked at me and screamed, "You're not even listening, you don't care." To which I calmly replied, "You're right. I am done."

Those five words put me in action to leave a relationship that was hurting and suppressing me. Five words, five seconds that made a solid decision in my brain. That small action put me in motion and changed the direction of my life.

Since then, I have become a cyclist, bodybuilder, and author. I fell in love with a man that respects and adores me, and we are building the life of our dreams. A life that wouldn't have happened had it not been for those few seconds of action.

Another time I took action was when I hired an editor for my first book about surgical menopause. *Come Back Strong: Balanced Wellness after Surgical Menopause* is part memoir and part self-help about my experience with hysterectomy and oophorectomy and my journey back to joy.

From this small step, my editor and I set a date to finish writing, the time frame for editing, and a plan to publish. My first book was published in November 2017.

Dreams come true when we take action.

Begin Again. Success Is Not Final

With purpose comes clarity. For every sixteen-week challenge I complete, I consider the end a beginning and I start again, knowing there are new goals to reach and new lessons to learn.

Whether you are starting a diet or exercise program, writing your first book, pursuing a dream or passion, improving your finances, or even embarking on a new relationship, courage is the step that moves you to action. It's human nature to struggle with procrastination from time to time. It's easy to say, "I'll start tomorrow, or Monday, or when I'm less busy or stressed."

Sometimes you may put things off because you simply don't feel like doing them. The reality is, if you wait until you feel like it, you may never get anything done.

Once you've taken the first step, momentum takes over as a powerful force that keeps you moving in the direction of your goals. Newton's first law of motion states that "An object at rest stays at rest and an object in motion stays in motion with the same speed and in the same direction unless acted upon by an unbalanced force."[14]

A commitment to finish is what will see you accomplish your goals every single time. So many people quit before they ever come close to reaching their goals.

There have been many times I've told someone I'm writing a book, and have been met with the response that they want to do that someday too. They may even start but years later, they are no closer to finishing it.

As I noted previously, in 2017, over 109,000 people started a sixteen-week challenge. Only 35,000 finished. Just 32% of the people that started the challenge actually completed it.

It takes courage to get started.

It takes discipline to consistently work toward your goal

Most of all, it requires a commitment to not only start on the path to success but commit to seeing it all the way to fruition. It takes a mindset to commit to finish. So much of the stress you feel isn't from your calendar being too full. It's from not finishing what you started. There were plenty of sixteen-week challenges where I wasn't making progress. There were times I was tempted to quit and start over, but I knew that would not serve me. That would be playing small. I stayed committed to finish what I started. Was the finished product what I had hoped for? No, but as they say in racing, "dead last is greater than did not finish (DFN), which trumps did not start (DNS)." Simply completing something I said I would do felt amazing and helped to propel me forward in the long run.

Whatever the goal you have for yourself, embrace the courage to start and the discipline to keep going. Take daily consistent action and commit to finishing, not simply starting. Continue to create healthier habits. Make decisions that move you toward your goals. Persist until you succeed. Always keep the promises you make to yourself. The practice of these skills is what will bring you success.

Wherever you are on your journey to success, I encourage you to continue toward your goal and dream. Become your best. Practice with consistency. Surround yourself with greatness and be quick to cooperate. Know that failure is a natural step in the process. Stay determined. Work with others in a spirit of collaboration, knowing that success loves company.

Remember that success is never a straight line, it's filled with peaks and valleys. It ebbs and flows with the seasons of your life. Make a deliberate effort to build the mindset to change your body and your life.

It's your turn to create your own transformation success story.

YOUR TURN

What are some of the promises you have made to others? Did you keep them?

_____

What are some of the promises you have made to yourself? Did you keep them?

_____

What thoughts or negative voices in your head do you need to let go of?

_____

What thoughts or positive voices in your head do you need to embrace?

_____

What action or aspect of transformation will you begin today?

_____

Notes

1. Irina Bancos, M.D, "What is Serotonin?" Hormone Health Network, (accessed August 9, 2021), https://www.hormone.org/your-health-and-hormones/glands-and-hormones-a-to-z/hormones/serotonin.
2. Crystal Raypole, "How to Hack Your Hormones for a Better Mood," Healthline, (accessed August 9, 2021), https://www.healthline.com/health/happy-hormone.
3. Jennifer Berry, "Endorphins: Effects and How to Increase Levels," Medical News Today, (accessed August 9, 2021), https://www.medicalnewstoday.com/articles/320839
4. Markus MacGill, "What is the link between love and oxytocin?" Medical News Today, (accessed August 9, 2021), https://www.medicalnewstoday.com/articles/275795.
5. Consumer Reports, "How Many Calories Are in Thanksgiving Dinner?" Consumer Reports, (accessed August 9, 2021), https://www.consumerreports.org/diet-nutrition/calories-in-your-thanksgiving-dinner/.
6. Wing, R. R. & Phelan, S. Am. J. Clin. Nutr. 82, 222S–225S (2005).
7. Mel Robbins, *The 5 Second Rule: Transform Your Life, Work, And Confidence With Everyday Courage* (n.p., Savio Republic, 2017), p. 35.
8. Og Mandino, *The Greatest Salesman in the World* (n.p., Bantam, 1985), p. 64.
9. Charles F. Haanel, "Part Four," The Master Key System: Your Step-by-Step Guide to Using the Law of Attraction (New York: Jeremy P. Tarcher, 2007), para. 12. Originally published as a correspondence course in 1912, and then as a book in 1917.
10. Debbie Ford, *Courage: Overcoming Fear and Igniting Self-Confidence*, (n.p., HarperOne, 2014), p. 61.
11. Marianne Williamson, *A Return to Love: Reflections on the Principles of A Course in Miracles,* (n.p., HarperSpotlight, 1993), p. 188.
12. Marianne Williamson, *A Return to Love: Reflections on the Principles of A Course in Miracles,* (n.p., HarperSpotlight, 1993), pp. 188-189.
13. Og Mandino, *The Greatest Salesman in the World* (n.p., Bantam, 1985), p. 70.

14. "Newton's First Law," The Physics Classroom, (accessed August 9, 2021),

15. https://www.physicsclassroom.com/class/newtlaws/Lesson-1/Newton-s-First-Law

Resources

Website

www.LoriAnnKing.com

Books By Lori Ann King

Come Back Strong: Balanced Wellness after Surgical Menopause

Wheels to Wellbeing: A Practical Self-Care Guide to Living a More Balanced Life

Courses by Lori Ann King

Balanced Wellness During Menopause

Books by Jim and Lori Ann King

Raging Love: An athlete's Journey to Self-Validation and Purpose (2022)

About the Author

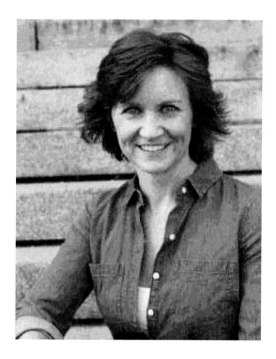

LORI ANN KING is on a mission to inspire you to live a life of true health, love, laughter, and freedom. She is the Amazon best-selling author of *Come Back Strong, Balanced Wellness After Surgical Menopause*, and a two-time contributor to the *Chicken Soup for the Soul* series.

Lori is a cyclist and was a runner for over twenty-five years, competing in races ranging in length from two to 26.2 miles. She is a 2019 IsaBody Challenge Finalist and 2017 IsaBody Honorable Mention. She has an undergraduate degree in Recreation from Western State College of Colorado and an advanced certificate in Information Management from Syracuse University.

When she's not writing, you'll find her with her husband, Jim on their bikes, paddleboards, kayaks, or in the gym.